ESSENTIALS OF
ART THERAPY TRAINING
AND PRACTICE

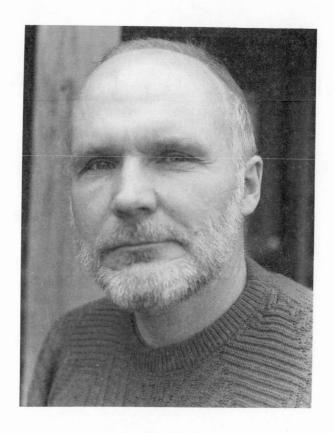

ABOUT THE AUTHOR

Bruce L. Moon is Director of the Clinical Internship in Art Therapy and the Clinical Art Therapy Graduate Intensive summer program at Harding Hospital, Worthington, Ohio. He is Chief of Adjunctive Therapy for the Child and Adolescent Division of Harding and an Adjunct Faculty Member of Lesley College. He has lectured and led workshops at many sites throughout the country.

Bruce is an active painter and poet-songwriter. He and his wife Cathy built their own log home in the country outside Columbus, Ohio, where they live with their children, Jesse and Brea, to whom this book is dedicated.

He brings to the profession a rich tradition of training in art education, theology and art therapy. The integration of these with his interests in existential philosophy, depth psychology, clinical work and training provides an intriguing, poetic and theoretical approach to art therapy training and practice.

ESSENTIALS OF ART THERAPY TRAINING AND PRACTICE

By

BRUCE L. MOON, M.A.C.E., M.Div., A.T.R.

Director, Clinical Internship in Art Therapy
Harding Hospital
Worthington, Ohio

With a Foreword by

James Lantz, Ph.D.

And an Introduction by

Catherine M. Moon, A.T.R

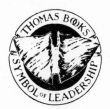

CHARLES C THOMAS • PUBLISHER
Springfield • Illinois • U.S.A.

Published and Distributed Throughout the World by

CHARLES C THOMAS • PUBLISHER
2600 South First Street
Springfield, Illinois 62794-9265

© *1992 by* CHARLES C THOMAS • PUBLISHER
ISBN 0-398-05794-X
Library of Congress Catalog Card Number: 92-3779

With THOMAS BOOKS *careful attention is given to all details of manufacturing
and design. It is the Publisher's desire to present books that are satisfactory as to their
physical qualities and artistic possibilities and appropriate for their particular use.*
THOMAS BOOKS *will be true to those laws of quality that assure a good name
and good will.*

Printed in the United States of America
SC-R-3

Library of Congress Cataloging-in-Publication Data

Moon, Bruce L.
    Essential of art therapy training and practice / by Bruce L. Moon ;
with a foreword by James Lantz ; and an introduction by Catherine M.
Moon.
        p.   cm.
    Includes bibliographical references and index.
    ISBN 0-398-05794-X
    1. Art therapy—Study and teaching.   2. Art therapy.   I. Title.
RC489.A7M659   1992
615.8'5156—dc20

                                                        92-3779
                                                        CIP

FOREWORD

Bruce Moon is an artist, a psychotherapist, an art therapist and a teacher of existential art therapy. Moon challenges the common attitude that the psychotherapist should be trained to be a technical practitioner whose interpretations are based upon cookbook prescriptions that are designed to confront psychopathology or maladaptive behavior, without understanding the personhood of the one who comes in pain to ask for the therapist's help.

Central to Moon's approach is the manner in which the mentor and the beginning art therapist come together in their efforts to learn and grow. Moon demonstrates the deep, intimate, alive and complex training relationship that can lead to the awareness of meaning in the lives of both. The concern for authentic engagement in the training relationship enhances the beginner's ability to use the *self* to help clients learn to use art and artistic expression to identify and integrate new insights in their lives.

Bruce's excellent book is ultimately concerned with the use of art and the artistic relationship to promote human growth. His deep understanding of both art and existentialism makes this book a high point in the ever-evolving fields of existential psychotherapy and art therapy. It is an important contribution to the development of creative, effective psychotherapists who value human growth and who refuse to slide into the dehumanizing trends of modern society. I highly recommend this book for those who are interested in art, art therapy, existential psychotherapy and the development of a future generation of psychotherapists who will dare to be creative, continuing to cherish the caring core of the helping process.

JIM LANTZ, PH.D.
Ohio State University and
Worthington Logotherapy Center

INTRODUCTION

At the close of one chapter in this book, Bruce says, "Attend to your passions. If you have lost the zeal that once powered your journey, return to the studio, for it is there that you first stumbled upon the power of images and art processes." If there is one essential element to this book on the essentials of art therapy, it is that art must be respected as the core of our profession. He does not suggest that we value the *art* above the *therapy*, but rather that to be an art therapist means there is no way to tease out one from the other. An art therapist who is "passionately disciplined" is willing to plunge into the dark depths of the soul and use what is found there as the very stuff of his or her art making. It is this fierce faith in the process of art making that undergirds our profession. This is what, at the most essential level, we art therapists bring to the patient-therapist and educator-student relationships.

With this "passionate discipline" as the warp that holds together the weft of his book, Bruce goes on to enumerate the various elements necessary for the training and practice of art therapists. His experience as an artist/clinician/educator gives the book credibility. He is not speaking theoretically about the necessary intertwining of these disciplines. He speaks with the voice of one actively engaged in these three aspects of art therapy. So it is that he can make assertions such as:

> Educators of art therapists must resist the seduction of training their students to be *as-if* psychologists or pseudo-psychiatrists.
> Students who want to become art therapists must insist that they be trained as art therapists and nothing less.
> If we abandon the art process for ourselves, we art therapists will eventually dry up and be blown away like dust.

Although you, as reader, may not agree with all that Bruce writes, it must be appreciated that he writes from the vantage point of one who lives his words. For this reason, what you read in this book may at times comfort, at times irritate, at times challenge and at times inspire you.

I think Bruce would say this is how it must be. It is not easy to be an art therapist, to be passionately disciplined. It is comforting, irritating, challenging, inspiring work. Bruce writes, "The work of the artist is not easy, covered with blisters both physical and emotional, tired muscles, cramped fingers and weary eyes. The work of an artist is a testament to faith that the struggle was worth it, that it mattered." If we art therapists bring this kind of faith to our work as educators and therapists, the clients we work with are sure to reap the benefits.

CATHERINE M. MOON, A.T.R.

PREFACE

In 1989 the membership of the American Art Therapy Association voted to alter the standards for registration by requiring a Masters Degree. I participated in the debates on this issue, both in public forums and through the AATA newsletter. I was, and am, concerned that the focus of discussion about the Masters requirement was most often centered on professional image, prestige, and licensure eligibility. Seldom did I hear or read that the well-being of clients would be much affected. It is my hope that patients will be the ultimate beneficiaries of more stringent educational requirements. If, as a side benefit, art therapists find that it is easier for them to be licensed or that they are held in higher esteem by professional colleagues, so much the better.

The debate has pushed me to examine what I believe to be the essential elements of art therapy training. As Director of the Clinical Internship in Art Therapy at Harding Hospital, I am in the unique position of being an educator, primary supervisor, program director as well as provider of fifteen hours of art psychotherapy clinical services per week. Through these different responsibilities I have an opportunity to observe and influence the training process. I am an advocate for the patient, the student, the faculty and the institution.

Selection of the title for this book, *Essentials of Art Therapy Training and Practice,* reflects my efforts to explore the crucial components of the education of creative arts therapists. The book was born of my desire to describe what I and my colleagues do as we integrate the complex fields of art, therapy and education. I hope to articulate clearly the elements of art therapy and art therapy training that are essential to the success of the student and practitioner. Whether we are successful with our students will one day affect the lives of the patients who come to them seeking help.

Over the past seventeen years I have worked with patients through music, drama, creative writing and sculpture, but it is in painting and drawing that I feel most comfortable. Therefore I will refer often to the visual arts experiences of patients and students. I hope that readers who specialize in other media will bear with me. While I embrace and appreciate the use of all of the creative arts, I am *at home* in the visual medium.

In writing, I have drawn from the experiences of the experts in the field of art therapy training: my students. I have asked them to teach me and I am grateful that they have been willing to do so. Their candor has allowed me to get as close to their experience as possible. They have even allowed portions of their daily journals to be shared here. Much of this work is also built around my interactions with the interns I supervise. Without the contributions of interns over the years, my understanding of the essentials of art therapy training would never have taken form.

This book is also about the practice of art therapy. It is impossible to write about training without reference to the clinical work that students are in training to do. Likewise, it would be difficult to write about the practice of art therapy without regard to the educational experiences that precede it. These two subjects are tightly interwoven, so I have integrated them in this book.

BRUCE L. MOON

AUTHOR'S NOTE

The clinical accounts in this book are in spirit true. In all instances, however, names have been changed and identifying information regarding patients has been so obscured as to insure the privacy and confidentiality of the persons with whom I have worked.

The case illustrations presented are amalgamations of many specific situations. Factual data has been fictionalized in order to protect the individual.

ACKNOWLEDGMENTS

I am indebted once again to many people who have, in their ways, contributed to the writing of this book. Special thanks go to Ellie Jones, my editor and colleague. She has worked wonders, smoothing and trimming my sometimes awkward presentation. She has also endured the rigors of reading my handwritten first drafts. Thanks also go to the contributors to this work, Jim Lantz, Catherine Moon, Deb DeBrular, Joan Selle and Lou Powers.

I've been deeply affected these past seventeen years by the creative, conflicted, painful and pleasurable encounters with my colleagues at Harding Hospital. I must also acknowledge the support I have received from the hospital administration. They've been interested, encouraging and, most important, they gave me time to write.

Finally, I want to thank the interns and patients I've come to know these past seventeen years. They are the ones who taught me most of what I believe to be the essentials of art therapy training and practice.

CONTENTS

ESSENTIALS OF
ART THERAPY TRAINING
AND PRACTICE

Chapter I

THE IMAGE

"Images and metaphors present themselves always as living psychic subjects with which I am obliged to be in relation ... A particular image is a necessary angel waiting for a response. How we greet this angel will depend on our sensitivity to its reality and presence."[1]

James Hillman, *The Blue Fire*

"Those who will not slip beneath
　　the still surface on the well of grief
turning downward through its black water
　　to the place we cannot breathe
will never know the source from which we drink
　　the secret water, cold and clear,
nor find in the darkness glimmering
　　the small round coins
　　　thrown by those who wished for something else."
David Whyte, *Where Many Rivers Meet*[2]

I would like to turn our attention to the place of *the image* in our profession. Although absolutely central to the existence of the creative arts therapies, it has received less attention in published works than one would expect. Authors seem comfortable describing art processes, art-making materials and tools, and of course art products. However, the image has received relatively little press. When image has taken center stage, it has often been in the service of a fixed scheme or theory. This does not, in my view, give image its proper respect. Image has been pressed, pounded or poured into an intellectual framework of under-standing generally related to interpretation. From such efforts come interpretive equations such as *that* means *that,* or *this* equals *this.* Invariably these cookbook engagements with image focus on pathology or illness, leading to a rather sick view of imagery. The works become popular because they reduce or eliminate ambiguity. They give the pretense of precision and promise a quantifiable result.

The reader of this text must abandon all hope of arriving at a systematic, verifiable formula for understanding the image. In my first book I coined the term *imagicide,* the killing of image.[3] We must avoid external pressures that would turn us into imagicidal practitioners. The first essential of the arts therapies is that we must regard images as living things. Whatever the form—the words of a poet, the tones of the musician, the brushstrokes of the painter or the fleeting gestures of dance—the image has a life (Fig. 1).

I have often argued that all things we create are self-portraits. As a result of my own evolution as an artist, I need to amend this argument. I still contend that all things I create are a self-portrait, but I now know that there is more to the image than just me.

In a lecture to the students of the Clinical Art Therapy Graduate Intensive at Harding Hospital, Shaun McNiff used the metaphor of children to demonstrate this point. While certainly our children reflect the characteristics of their parents, he insisted, children are *not* their parents. "They have a life of their own."[4] As a parent, I know he is right.

I have often referred to H. W. Janson's description of art making as a birth process.[5] So, if the image I release upon the canvas may be likened to my child, I am forced to modify my previous conviction that it is no more than a portrait of me. My real-life children remind me constantly that they are not me. When I look at the images in my art I am confronted with this same reality. I must speak to my painting respectfully, regarding it as both me and not me.

The notion that image has a life of its own and its own stories to tell can be demonstrated at an art exhibit. Ask the viewers of any piece to tell the story of the work and be intrigued by what will emerge! Compared with the comments told by the artist/creator, no two stories are exactly the same.

I admire the work of Edward Hopper and one of my favorites is his painting, *Nighthawks.*[6] I have never read a description by Hopper of his intent with this painting. I have actually avoided doing so. The stories this image tells me are far more interesting to me than any he may have written or spoken of. The painting has a life of its own, separate and distinct from that of Edward Hopper. To be sure, I believe that it may represent many facets of Hopper the man, but it represents itself to me

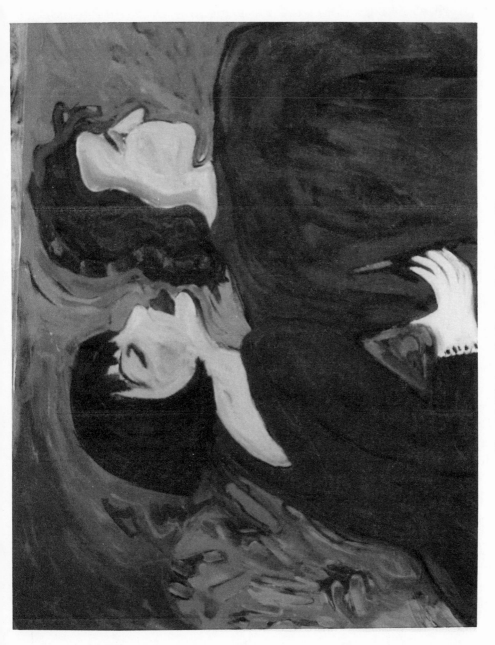

Figure 1. Whatever the form . . . the image has life.

without his intrusion. In the words of Hillman, it is a necessary angel awaiting my response to its message.

In April of 1991 I was a consultant to the Midwestern Illinois Arts Therapy Conference hosted by Jerilee Cain, Ph.D., at Western Illinois University. The keynote speaker was David Whyte, a poet from the Pacific northwest. During his presentation he recited his poem, *The Well of Grief.* As his resonant voice rose, I was caught up in wonder. " . . . in the darkness glimmering, the small round coins thrown by those who wished for something else."[2]

I have no idea what personal pain Whyte's words represent, but I have a very clear image of myself lying deep in the murky well waters as the shiny slivers of another's wishes tumble past. I recall the faces of grief I have known. I remember the tugging, gnawing, longing to be on the surface, away from my own mourning. David Whyte's image " . . . glimmering, the small round coins . . . "[2] becomes my image. A necessary angel, it waits for my response. It will not leave me alone. It calls me into dialogue. I speak with the image and it teaches me, not only about David Whyte, but about myself as well.

To regard the image as being greater than, or more than a reflection of the self who created it requires a willingness to let go. I can best explain this by referring to my own art work. The painting in Figure 2 is of the little cafe in my hometown where my friends and I gathered throughout my adolescence. I painted it during a period of intense reflection and introspection about my past. It is one of a series of paintings with similar themes, that is, scenes of my childhood. When I look at this painting I can smell the hamburgers and fries, I can hear the laughter of my buddies. I remember standing on the corner, heartbroken after breaking up with my girlfriend. I remember the feel of sitting in the 1965 VW beetle that is parked beside the building.

These memories and sensations are rich and meaningful for me. However, when I recently exhibited the painting in the Harding Hospital auditorium, I was fascinated by the comments others made about it. Each viewer made up his or her own story to fit the scene. Of course none of their stories matched my own. There was a moment of artist-indignation as I eavesdropped on others' reactions to the work, but it became clear that the stories others told about this image had some personal meaning to the storyteller. My painting called them into a dialogue that was different from the one I experienced. I began to understand the meaning of letting go. I could not control how the image conversed with someone

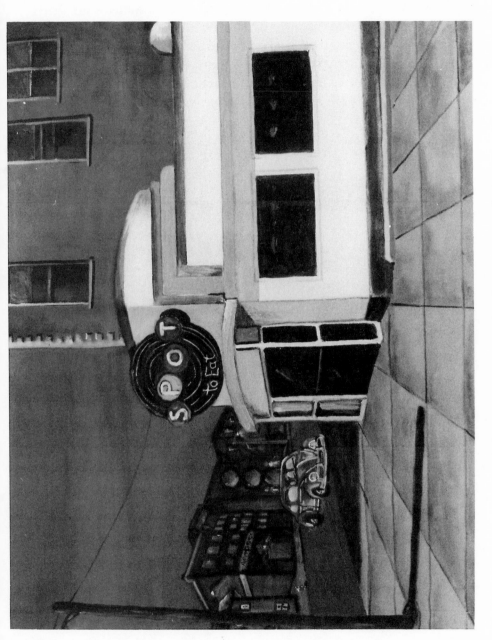

Figure 2. Each viewer made up his or her own story to fit the scene.

else. The image asserted its own existence. Had I intervened and said, "No, you misunderstand . . . this painting is about . . ." I would have committed imagicide (and perhaps symbolic infanticide as well). All I could do was let go.

Catherine Moon describes this process of hearing others dialogue with her images as like trying on someone else's perspective.[7] It is instructive, for it deepens and expands the artist's own dialogue with the work (Fig. 3).

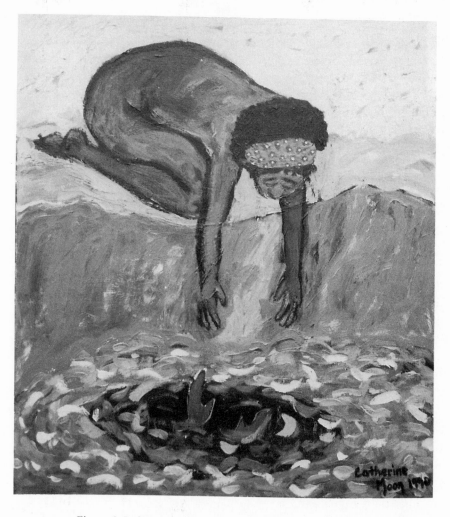

Figure 3. It deepens and expands the artists own dialogue.

Those who use a classic psychoanalytic theoretical framework would classify these encounters as *projections*. I do not object to this description if projection is seen as the cornerstone of empathy and not as a building block of pathology. I believe that ultimately it is the ability of the creative arts therapist to project one's self into the image of the patient, laying the groundwork for the establishment of a therapeutic relationship. It can be argued that all good relationships are formed through disciplined acknowledgment of and willingness to work with mutual projective experiences. This suggests that art and life imitate each other. Both are dynamic, moving and subject to change.

It could be formulized as follows: I project upon you, you project upon me and then we attempt to make sensible meaning out of the process.

This is a possible description of the interaction among the creative arts therapist, the patient/client and the image before them. The image is the intermediary. It is not only an object-thing to be used as the basis of patient revelatory conversation. It is a subject capable of teaching both patient and therapist about themselves and one another.

From this perspective one begins to view the image as a sacred, living thing. As arts therapists, then, we are those who attend to live images as well as to the living persons who made them.

I believe that Kirkegaard touches on such a perspective as he discusses devotional listening. "In a devotional sense, ... to listen in order to act, this is the highest thing of all, and, God be praised, every man is capable of it if he so wills."[8] I propose that we art therapists adopt the phrase *devotional seeing*. To see in order to act (the action being the attending to) and every art therapist is capable of it if he or she so wills.

Hyperattention to pathology has had a malevolent impact upon our ability to regard images and their creators as entities worthy of our respect.

I encourage the student reader and seasoned practitioner alike to stop looking for any formula or system for analyzing images, either your own or your patients'. You will never be able to establish that *this* always means *that*, or that $a+b=c$. The image cannot be measured or verified. It is not concrete. Images will always be ambiguous, precocious and subject to change. The world of imagery is full of shadow and mist, a spectrum of gray areas. Embrace the mystery. Dedicate yourself to devotional seeing and constant exploration in a world where nothing is sure.

The place of the image in the creative arts therapy professions is at the center . . . the heart. Enjoy your clumsy, stammering, stumbling attempts at dialogue. This is the essential nature of what we art therapists do.

Chapter II

BEGINNINGS

THE STORY OF IT
(A FAIRY TALE)

In a land known as Wo there lived a girl of fourteen summers. She was a kind and gentle girl, not beautiful, not ugly either. She was troubled, though. A question had arisen within her during the summer of her twelfth year, *What is the meaning of It?* Although she tried to put it out of her mind, the question would not go away. Every day, hundreds of times, she found herself wondering, *What does It mean?*

Oh, she knew that people said that it was too bad. Her mother, in an angry mood one day, said, "It is your father's fault." Her older brother told her it bugged him. Sometimes she overheard her aunts and uncles muttering that she would never make it. The only thing she didn't know was what it meant. The question haunted her day and night. Sometimes she would dream that she was opening a large box where it would be, but she always woke up too soon to see it.

During the summer of her fourteenth year she was so vexed by it that she decided at last she must do something. She decided to run away. She intended to ask everyone she met what was the meaning of it.

Finally, on the morning of the middle day of the middle month of the season, she crept out of her house and began her journey. Everywhere she went she asked the people she met what It meant. A constable told her it was the law. An athlete told her it was winning. A businessman told her it was profit, and two lovers told her it was just being together.

While all these answers seemed plausible enough, somehow for her they just didn't seem quite right. And so she traveled and asked, walked and listened, but was never satisfied. At long last, worn out and feeling defeated, she decided to return home. That night as she slept, she had a dream.

In the dream she had walked across a desert and was very, very thirsty. She came upon a shimmering lake. She knelt down on the bank and tried to scoop some water with one hand. She had to be cautious, for she could not swim and she wasn't sure how deep the water was. The wanderer was so thirsty, but each time she tried to scoop water with her hand, it all ran out of her grasp before she could get it to her lips. In the dream she felt that she might die if she couldn't quench her thirst.

Suddenly an old woman appeared on the bank beside her. The old woman had long silvery hair and was dressed in a blue cloak. She reached out and gently touched the girl's shoulder. "You must use both hands," she said. The girl shuddered, "But I might fall in and drown!" The old woman sat quietly for a bit, then said, "You may die of thirst or die of drowning. I tell you, you must decide to risk."

The girl's throat was parched and she longed for the cool relief. "Couldn't you help me?" The old woman frowned, then gently sighed, "I am not thirsty. You must decide. That is all there is to it." With that, she disappeared.

***

Students come to training seeking the meaning of It for their lives. With them they bring all the answers they have been given throughout their history. They bring volumes of questions, mental cassette tapes full of self-definitions and catalogues of how they think the world should be. As the mentor, it is your task to help them question their answers, answer their questions, edit, delete and re-record their self-definitions, and expand their repertoire of ideas, feelings and values in relation to how the world is.

JOURNEY

Mary Lou Powers

Sometime in the middle of August, 1985, I was in my classroom at the Columbus College of Art and Design, where I taught undergraduate courses in Introduction and Advanced theory and methods in Art Therapy. The college hosts an annual open house at which instructors from all the various divisions give presentations or lead discussions about their specialty areas. On this particular evening I was surprised by the appearance in my room of Mary Lou (Stith) Powers. I had known Lou for several years. She was, and still is, a teacher specializing in educating severely learning handicapped children and adolescents in the on-campus school at Harding Hospital.

Our paths had crossed professionally from time to time, but we had not gotten along very well. My impressions of Lou were that she was rather hostile, liked to be in charge. She seemed challenging in a devaluing way. Lou recalls that her initial views of me included perceptions that I was chauvinistic, overly competitive, flamboyant and controlling. In short, neither of us cared much for the other. Therefore I was somewhat uneasy when, after hearing my presentation about my courses, Lou informed me that she intended to register for the advanced theory and methods class.

I worried about how she would fit in with a class of college sophomores and juniors. Lou already had nearly twenty years' teaching experience. Obviously, she would be at a very different level than her fellow students. I also worried that she might be difficult to deal with in class. I had heard from colleagues at the hospital of her reputation for assertive critical engagement in meetings. I wondered if I was competent to teach a woman like Lou.

The semester opened three weeks after the open house. True to her word, Lou sat in the front row of the class. There was no escape. I had to establish a relationship with her. We began.

My first lecture to every class begins, "All things we create are a self-portrait."[3] In my ruminations on my fears about Lou's participation in the class, I had failed to have faith in the awesome power of the art process. In the thirty-two weeks that followed the first class, Lou painted

13

and drew and scribbled portraits of herself as I had never imagined her. Perhaps most poignant was a drawing that depicted herself as having an outer layer of rhinocerous skin that concealed and protected her real doeskin. Images of a broken marriage, a troubled son, an ill brother and a vulnerable self emerged. Our relationship transformed from a dance reminiscent of heavyweight boxers circling and measuring one another, to a rather awkward ballet. In the midst of our unfolding relationship, Lou began to ask questions about the Clinical Internship in Art Therapy. Near the end of her second semester she applied for appointment to the Internship and was accepted for entry the following fall.

The initial educational plan designed for Lou focused on four primary components:

First, since Lou came to the program with vast experience as a teacher with adolescents, we agreed to provide her with clinical exposure to adult patients in the hospital. Her original schedule included an exercise (physical conditioning) group, horticulture therapy, an adult expressive arts psychotherapy group, and creative arts studio. She was also assigned to be a psychiatric team member on a long term adult unit.

Second, the faculty was concerned that Lou's engagement with and knowledge of visual arts media was rather weak. It was decided that she would be urged in the creative arts studio to explore a variety of fine arts modalities, among them painting, drawing and sculpture.

Third, Lou was entered into the Philosophy of Art Therapy Seminar and the Art Therapy Interns Process Group. The focus was to be the development of a personal philosophy of treatment, with opportunities for experimental implementation and integration of the clinical experiences she would have.

Finally, she was assigned an individual supervisor/mentor who would serve as her guide through the training process.

A cornerstone of the mentor-intern relationship is the intern's journal. The journal is to be written on a daily basis and is to reflect the journey of the student through the training process. The journal is often a sketch book as well, chronicling in words and pictures the intensity of the educational experience. The interns are given very few guidelines for the journal. All they are told is that it is to be kept current and that it will be read by the supervisor on a weekly basis.

To help the reader to understand the early stages of the art therapy educational journey, the following excerpts from Lou's journal are offered.

Names of patients and student peers have been changed for purposes of confidentiality (Fig. 4).

6/20   Bruce asks
But why do we do art?
I don't understand "soul"
Art proclaims, I AM, I AM
What about the dignity of man?

6/21   —stretch—
pull gently
Bandana Lady!
"Can I love you"
You don't scare me!
I've seen your pain
Relationship. . . .
Relationship. . . .
Relationship. . . .
Process . . . Climb the mountain

6/23   A whole week here. I love it.
No fussing about being therapeutic.
Imagine.

INTERN PROCESS GROUP:
    Young, your scab.
    All nervous, excited
    It's out there.
    Mysterious Dana
    Who says one thing but secrets another
    And dear Josh
    Caren, I'm glad you're here!
Completed flower drawing. It's good.
Adults are just adolescents
in grownup bodies
The tasks are the same!

6/24   Dear Bruce,
    Why do I do art?
    Because you say, do art.
    Once long ago I did art
    because *I* had to, perhaps
    I'll rediscover that person.

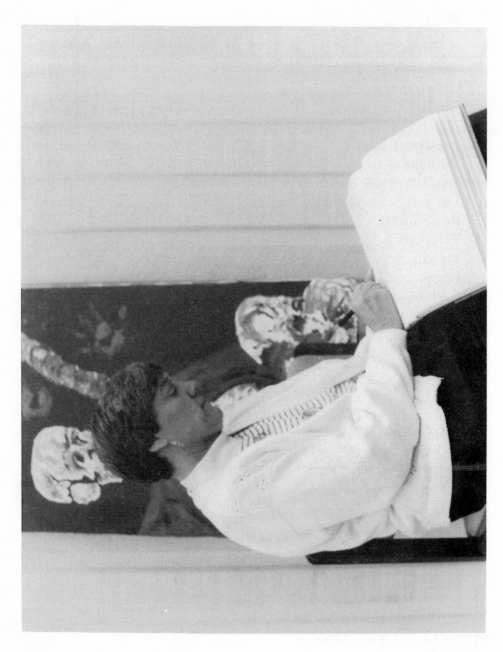

Figure 4. Why do I do art?

One thing is for sure
I do therapy because I
have to, it swells inside
and bubbles out.

ARPS HALL

A visit to the library
reaffirms my quest
I know that if I don't
continue to learn and study
and grow
I'll go stagnant.

6/26

I feel more in the flow
I gave Laurie a tour of the school—
So much of my ego still there.
Wanted to join Ruth, Ali and Gail today
Perhaps adults are important too—
I always thought kids were the main
focus of my energies.
Oh, Barri! so young, so full of life—
What joy to share this time with you.
How short the time is.
A pressing need to *know* all.
Where will this lead?

6/28   Working with the adjunctive therapy
staff is a real treat.
I experience none of the crazy
hostile feeling, Why?
Truly a nurturing staff. I'm able
to let the doeskin show.
We had lunch at a chinese place
Wonderful—I'm reconnecting with
Andy B., it's been years.
J. shared her eating disorder with me.
I'd shared my L.D. problems in group
with her.
My name tag says
    Lou Powers, A. T.

6/29   I'm painfully aware of how short my
time is.
My worst fantasy has come true,
I love this.
Why do I do art?
Because Bruce says, "Draw"
and I can find parts of my
youth in the task.
I experience total absorption
but will I continue to draw?
Who knows?
Why do therapy.
Because I can't not do therapy.
It flows from within,
not to do it is to die.
PROCESS GROUP:
Deb asked again if I was protecting Josh.
I hope not, the pain will be suffered.
Perhaps it's my effort to join his journey.
If he won't come to us, admit membership
Then I'll go to him.
Dana—finally her affect fit her voice.
I struggle to include Jan, but am
certainly aware that she is an outsider.
The experience is not the same for her.
Caren continues to look brighter, more
confident in herself.
I hope I shared the pain of David,
the years of doubt.

7/4   Perhaps I'm finding the artist in me.
It was there at one time, adolescence.
Cathy Moon's suggestion that I selected
art therapy for a reason must be true.
Thank you.
My research in sexual abuse confirms
what I've been seeing in the
adolescent population here.
More abused kids, both male and female.
Generational abuse

relationship between abuse and
self-mutilation.

7/5   I was very anxious in research group. Probably because
of Caren. My topic, sexual abuse, is a good one
considering the number of patients we serve with this
problem, but my knowledge of her abuse made it harder.
I don't want to leak this information to the group
members, but let Caren tell it in her own time. I was
angry when Deb pushed her.
Counter-transference issues may remind me of
my own passivity? Perhaps, what willing victims we
all were—(women)
I was upset that my art might be uninteresting. The artist is alive.

7/7   Judy and I had a terrific expressive art group. We
seem to work so well together. An extra pair of
ears and eyes. What a nice flow. I really respect
her and feel that she respects me too.
We have shared issues and concerns. This feels right.
What about relationship is so scary?
She talked about controlling relationship
Ending when she can't be in charge.
How can someone love me after all that
I've been through.
If I pull the bandage off to make myself
vulnerable, I risk losing a friend—it's
painful, especially if I value friendship
more than they do.
PROCESS GROUP
    Some in the group see Bruce and Deb
    as authority figures.
    Josh continues to distance himself
    Caren and I had a mini after-group
    discussion, just comforting and
    acknowledging Josh's pain and
    our support of him.

7/13   I must put limits on D.
She is very devaluing.
How hard this seems to be
compared to adolescents.

I've set limits with her before,
so I will again.
I need to explore fantasy in
expressive arts group. I want
to let patients know my world.
So many questions about Josh.
Obviously he is very frightened
of intimacy.
I just want his friendship,
not his body. I guess I'll
never know.
Bruce—I bought two blank canvases.
What about that?

7/19 I've been neglectful of this
journal process.
I started painting today.
It felt good
    mixing colors
    putting brush to canvas
    in my mind's eye I have
    an image
    perhaps my hand will create this.
Jody, Caren and I chatted after work about art,
technique, process—
I actually sounded like I knew
what I was talking about.
Well, reading is my strong point.
We will see if my hand can
make what my eye has read.
I have never experienced such
acceptance and validation of
self-worth as I have this summer.
Even staff members whom I don't work
with have made positive comments.

7/25 Big thrill, but scary.
Jody wants me to lead her
expressive arts group while
she's on vacation. I'm on my own.

I feel more confident, stronger.
How good it is to be valued.

7/27   POEM

     My object is saddened, confused
     and empathic
     A sudden breeze
       will it spin . . . or fall
     Two pieces, yet one
       each unto itself.
     My journey has begun
     The risk must be taken
     From some protective mother's,
     brother's, lover's, father's arm
     On to wilderness, to change.
     Softness returns as red,
     raw violence abates.
     From pain and conflict
     to life and growth.

            Lou Powers[9]

In this slice of life, this quick glimpse of two months of Lou's inner commentary on her training to become an art therapist, we catch the shiny surfaces and treacherous shadows of her experience.

A recurring reference throughout Lou's journal is to my questioning her, "Why do you make art?" It reflects the major thrust of her experience in training. It is important to remember that Lou came to the program after nearly twenty years' experience in teaching learning disabled adolescents in a psychiatric setting. For her there was little or no question of her academic background or clinical/relationship skills. What Lou clearly lacked was, 1) an understanding of the visual arts language, and 2) a view of herself as an artist/therapist. For Lou's professional and personal growth, it was essential that she engage in a training program capable of flexing to meet her particular educational needs.

The development of one's own therapeutic style is a process as individual as one's own art products. As the professions of the creative arts therapies move into the 1990's and beyond, they must develop standards of education that are both meaningful and diverse.

Chapter III

BEGINNER'S CHAOS

Although students come to training with varied academic and personal histories, it is relatively safe to assume that the early stages of their journey are experienced as chaos. In our program we admit students who are fresh from undergraduate school as well as some who already hold an advanced degree in a related field. Some of our students are twenty-one years old, while others have been in their fifties and beyond. Some have had extensive psychological treatment experience; others have had little or no contact with the emotionally disturbed. One commonality is that beginning is a chaotic experience. As educators, we are behooved to remain aware of the disorientation that new environments, new expectations and new experiences can create (Fig. 5).

While every academic, institute and clinical training program has its own idiosyncrasies, there are general factors that lead to beginner's chaos. Among these are the realities of finding one's way around a new facility. In our particular setting this requires learning the names of fifteen buildings and their location on a fifty-acre campus. There are specific rooms and areas within each of these buildings. Some of the areas are open to public access, some require keys. Along with the geographical layout of the campus, students are quickly introduced to a host of individuals. They begin their relationship with their primary supervisor, they meet the faculty, their peers, adjunct personnel, and in our setting, patients. In addition they are quickly engaged in meetings where other unseen persons are referred to. Doctors, social workers, nurses, medical directors, psychologists, technicians, etc., etc. In the first week of training the student may encounter fifty or more people. This in itself can be overwhelming.

Another aspect of the chaos is that beginning training marks the end of anticipating, planning for future education. Most students have thought long and hard about their choice of careers. Many students have had to make sacrifices in order to be in training. Some have waited a long time between their initial decision to enter training and actually beginning

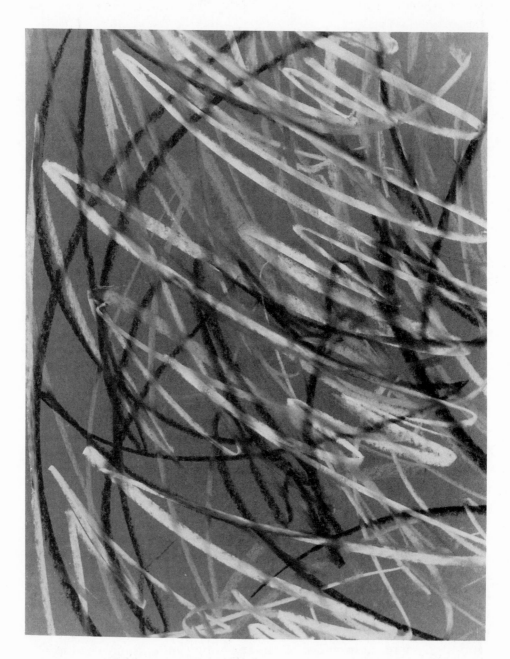

Figure 5. The early stages of their journey are experienced as chaos.

the process. These circumstances lead to internal anxiety as the training is begun.

Students also often struggle with their own doubts as they embark on this new phase of their lives. They are plagued by questions such as: *Is this what I really want to do? Do they like me? Am I really good enough to be successful here? What if I don't like it here after I've started?* Many old feelings of insecurity are stirred as the training starts.

Finally, add to this mix the mysterious nature of the creative arts therapy field itself, and we begin to glimpse the new students' internal experience as they take the first steps of their journey. It is as if their world were one of those glass balls with white flakes suspended in liquid. Entry into training to become an arts therapist is a little like shaking the glass, creating a snow storm. Yet, in most cases the flurry remains internal while the student's exterior appears smooth and undisturbed. Certainly no graduate student in any field wants to be seen as in turmoil. It is the responsibility of the faculty supervisor to be *tuned in* to the experience of the student.

The initial chaos of the student is ultimately necessary and of great benefit. It is necessary in that entry into training should be a fairly dramatic transitional period in the student's life. An old way of being is left behind while a new way is as yet unclear. As are all passages in life, this is accompanied with a measure of fear, excitement and anxiety.

It is of benefit to the student in that it presents him or her with a potent, double-edged metaphor that should become a powerful tool in both their educational pursuits and in their professional practice down the road.

One edge of this "beginner's chaos" metaphor is the art process itself. The sensitive educator will engage the student in this metaphor by discussing the parallels of beginning training and starting a new art work (Fig. 6). As the artist approaches the studio, the possibilities are endless. Countless subtle choices are made consciously and unconsciously. What medium will be used? In the case of a painting, what size and shape of canvas? What tools will be employed? Representational or non-representational? Abstract or highly rendered? Content? Color? Form? Shape? Emotional tone?.... and on and on. There are thousands, even millions of potential images that could emerge as the artist works. They make up the chaotic sea of possibilities. Each question the artist answers, each decision made as the work unfolds serves to bring structure and order to the chaos so that the artistic product can be realized. Perhaps the deepest sense of gratification and connection to our work that we artists can experience comes from this profound process of making order from disordered potential.

It is through the multiple decisions, subtle and overt, that the artist begins to uncover the essence of an art piece. This essential quality may never be put into words by the artist, yet it is comprehended at a deep level that is either pre- or meta-verbal.

The engagement in art processes is an enactment of one's potential to structure the chaos of multiple possibilities. This is exactly the same position in which the new trainees find themselves. The possibilities are numerous and at first seem confusing and jumbled. Some of their internal questions are, *Is this field valid? Which am I, artist or therapist? What is the most important—process or product? What kinds of patients do I want to work with? What will I do well? What if I do harm to someone? Why do I want to do this work?*

It is important, in all stages of training but particularly in the initial phases, to refer the student to the art process itself.

I have vivid recall of a student coming into my office for a supervisory session and slamming my door. She sat down and immediately poured out the anger she felt toward a psychiatrist who had made an offhanded devaluing comment about art therapy. He had referred to a group of which my student was a co-leader as "voodoo group." The psychiatrist's attempt at humor had pushed my student's buttons. I let her vent for a few minutes, then shifted the conversation towards a more detached observing-ego position. I suggested that we explore all the possible interpretations we could make of the psychiatrist's "voodoo" comment.

The student's anger rapidly dissolved into tears as she got in touch with her own feelings of inadequacy and doubts about the art therapy profession. Questions came so quickly, with no time for attempts at answers, that my supervisory role became that of an empathic listener. As the session neared its close there was still much to be addressed. I suggested that she spend some time in the studio making art.

The next morning I found three vivid drawings lying on a chair in my office (Fig. 7). The images were intense. The first was a tangled mass of color and line, reminiscent of a large pile of knotted yarn scraps. The second image utilized the same colors, but there was a vague hint of a facial form in the turmoil of lines. The third image was a self-portrait. The colors were consistent with those of the first two drawings and although there were still knots and tangles in the lines, the face was

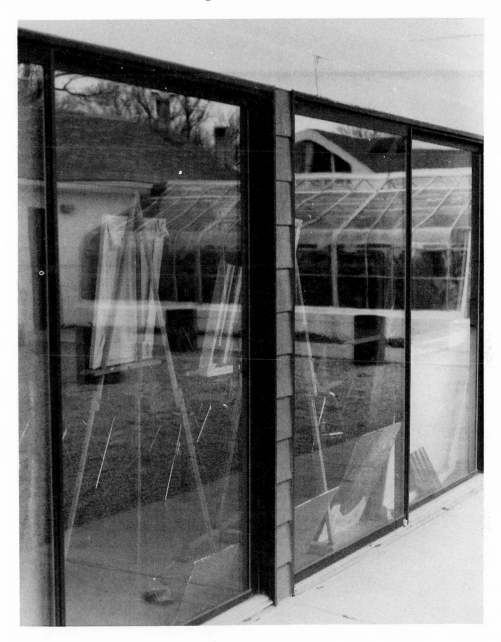

Figure 6. As the artist approaches the studio the possibilities are endless.

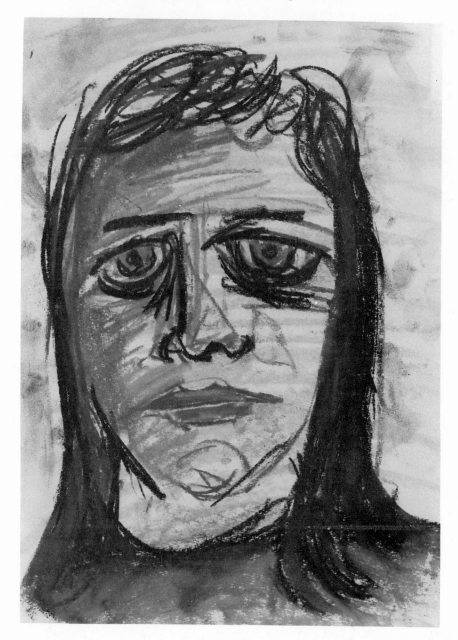

Figure 7. The colors were consistent with those of the first two drawings.

clearly represented. In an artistic sense the student had laid out the road map of her internal journey. These three drawings became our starting point for many supervisory sessions. What began as a jumbled, angry, hurt mass of colorful lines eventually formed a solid portrait. By the time her training ended, she was able to joke with the psychiatrist about the *voodoo* she does and the *art* of medicine that he practices.

The other edge of the beginner's chaos metaphor relates to the parallel between embarking on the training journey and the patient's experience in beginning treatment. The confusion, the pain, anxiety, excitement and fears generated in the student are a wonderful resource, for they connect the therapist-trainee with the patient's experience.

The longer an arts therapist practices, the harder it is to stay attuned to the internal turmoil of the patient. Doing art therapy is what is normal and routine for the art therapist. The awe inevitably diminishes as the therapist seasons. It is important to impress upon the student how similar are his or her fears, hopes, anxieties in beginning training to those of the patient entering treatment. It is a precious window into the world of the patient. The beginning student of course cannot know this. It must be interpreted as it is experienced in the present.

Chapter IV

THE JOURNEY METAPHOR IN TRAINING

The hero, whether of fairy tale, myth or movie, always begins the transformation from his ordinary life to his heroic life by embarking upon a journey. The quest is marked by encounters with agents of evil and good. It has pitfalls and terrible moments when the hero fears that his efforts have been folly and all is lost. The journey is sometimes a descent into the darkness of one's soul, where the engagements with powerful forces are not of the external sort, but rather the internal wrestlings of virtue and the vile. Ultimately the hero comes to terms with both the forces of his inner life and the powers of the world. Whether by killing, or taming or naming them, the hero emerges from the struggle forever changed (Fig. 8).

As I sit in my office at the hospital interviewing prospective students, I often think of the image of the hero. I try to tell them what a difficult and treacherous journey they are volunteering for. I speak of the stress of spending eight hours a day in an atmosphere that is often tense, painful and exhausting. I mention the constant stream of books and articles to be read, the papers to be researched and written. I tell stories about patients I have known, about their battered pasts, their abused childhoods, their shattered present and bleak future. I warn these would-be heroes of the strenuous physical schedule they will be expected to follow. And I tell them of the emotional calluses I've had to grow.

After all that, I talk about the joy of seeing a patient leave the hospital who has really made the sought-for gains. I speak of love and tenderness, spirit and art.

Some prospective students come to me as they are nearing the end of undergraduate careers in the fine arts, psychology or art education. Others are middle-aged, restless with their current professions, vaguely unhappy with the course their lives have taken. Their children are now in elementary school. They feel called to a different life. Still another group of wouldbe therapists already possess degrees from more traditional academic settings. They long for a more intense educational

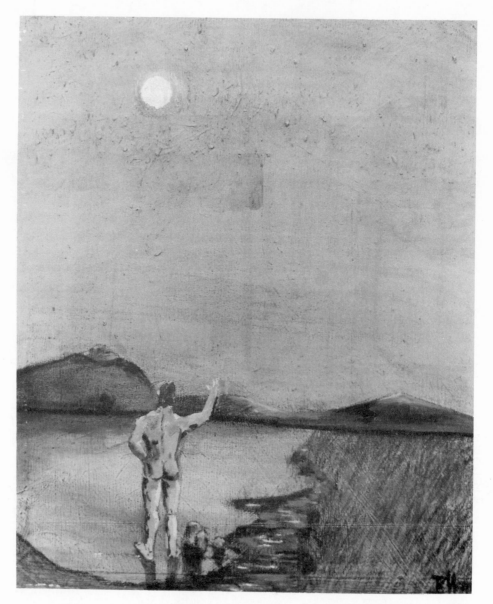

Figure 8. The quest is marked by encounters with agents of evil and good.

experience. Regardless of their age, background or motivations, I try to frame with them the concept of the heroic journey engendered by training to become a creative arts therapist.

The tightly intertwined phenomena of art, therapy and personal heroic quest form the foundation of the field. These processes swirl together and force tremendous demands upon the student. The individual is called to new levels of emotional, physical, cognitive and spiritual involvement in the struggle. The intensity of the journey led one of our recent interns, Darienne Veri, to exclaim, "It's not a normal life!" I could only agree that being a therapist is not a normal life, and surely being in the early stages of becoming one accentuates the abnormality. One must be ready and willing to go on a heroic journey.

Interns often begin their year-long quest with excitement and enthusiasm, not unlike the honeymoon and newlywed periods of marriage. It is fun. Everything is new and interesting. They are filled with energy. Very soon, however, their excitement encounters the powerful realities of patients in extreme emotional pain, with brutal histories and tragic experiences in the present. Enthusiasm is transformed into self-doubt, depression and confusion. Inevitably the student's comfortable self-image is challenged by deep intrapsychic stirrings.

Becoming a creative arts therapist requires an extraordinary willingness to introspect and struggle with the images one finds in the mirror. It is often quite difficult. The student who comes from a fine arts background at times sees the personal exploration and self-confrontation as intrusive and threatening to expressive freedom. With these students, the recurrent question, "Why do you make art?" is heard as an impingement on their creativity. Such a student lamented, "Why do I need to know? Isn't it enough that I *do* make art?"

To the intern who comes from a solid academic background, the making of self as the subject of inquiry is foreign. These students begin with the belief that all they need to know about a given subject must be written somewhere in the literature of the field. For them the first few steps of their heroic quest are filled with reluctance and concern. All novice art therapists must wrestle with a new mode of learning in which they are both subject and object of inquiry.

A STORY

In a certain tribe of nomads, it was the custom to send scouts into the desert to find water. For some time now, the scouts had been disappearing, and the chief was growing concerned. The tribe was beginning to question his wisdom in sending the men out. Yet, the chief knew that they must seek water. He began to send the scouts out two by two. They vanished. The next scouts went in parties of five. They, too disappeared without a trace. The situation was becoming critical, but the chief did not know what to do.

At about that time, a young would-be hero arrived at the tent village. He sought out the chief and told him he'd heard they were having some trouble. The chief explained the situation, adding that he was feeling quite desperate.

"Don't worry," said the young man, "I will go out into the desert for you, and I will find water."

The would-be hero left the village and struck out into the barren wilderness. When he reached a certain place, he found a large crack in the earth. A cold wind surged up from the darkness. For a moment the hero hesitated, then asked himself, "What in the world am I getting myself into? Why should I care if that tribe back there has water? This looks like a dangerous place" (Fig. 9).

As his doubts echoed within him, he began to back away from the crevice. The crack lengthened and followed him. The farther he withdrew, the closer came the cold darkness. He realized that if he turned and ran, he would be swallowed up. He stood paralyzed for several moments. Suddenly the wind gusted and sand swirled about him. A hooded figure appeared, shimmering in the blowing sand. It spoke.

"You must not run away from this place."

The hero replied, "But this is more than I bargained for. What can I do?"

Again the hooded figure spoke, "You must not run away, and you cannot stay where you are. The dilemma is your own."

With that, the figure disappeared into the sand.

The would-be hero did the only thing he could. He turned to face the darkness and slowly walked down through the opening. There he discovered a hidden river. On the far bank he saw the remains of the tribal scouts who had preceded him, who had tried to run from the darkness.

***

The process of becoming an art therapist continually challenges the defenses of the novice. There is a steady focus on the hidden underground rivers of the intern's life and the lives he comes into contact with. For many students, this is a period of unprecedented growth.

The success or failure of the journey depends upon the quality of the

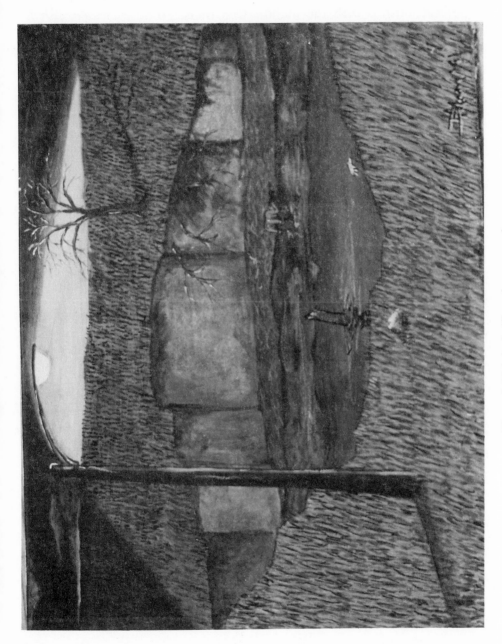

Figure 9. This looks like a dangerous place.

relationship between the student and the mentor/supervisor. While it is clearly the work of the intern that determines the outcome of the training, it is the relationship with the mentor that fuels, guides, corrects and consoles the apprentice in mid-journey.

Chapter V

THE MENTOR SUPERVISOR

I believe that one of the essential elements of an effective art therapy training experience is the Mentor/Supervisor relationship. To begin this exploration of supervision, I turned to the dictionary, which gives the definition, "the direction and critical evaluation of instruction."[5] the word is derived from the Latin *super* (over) and *videre* (to watch, to see). Therefore, a supervisor is "an overseer, one who watches over the work of another with responsibility for its quality."

This definition emphasizes the administrative functions of supervision, i.e., to see that the task is executed at acceptable quantitative and qualitative levels. As a supervisor and director of a training program, I must sometimes confront issues such as daily schedules, tardiness or misbehavior in the workplace; however, this type of administrative supervision is seldom used in my relationship with students in the clinical educational milieu.

A second aspect of supervision is the provision of education for the supervisee. Here the relationship is defined as a cooperative process through which the supervisor helps the supervisee to use the educational structure to gain the best possible learning experience. It is this function of supervision that is most often the focus of the relationship between student and instructor. It also responds to the student's desire for a relationship with someone who knows the answers.

While the first definition emphasizes the functional objectives of the training setting (administrative), the second emphasizes the cognitive development of the student (educational). Each of these descriptions is correct only in part. It is true that the creative arts therapy supervision is both an administrative and educational process. The experienced art therapy practitioner has responsibility for implementing both functions in working with students.

It is my sense that there is yet another markedly different responsibility that must be included in any definition of creative arts therapy supervision. This is the supportive, expressive role-modeling function of supervision. The supervisor has the responsibility to maintain intern morale, help with the inevitable discouragements and doubts that arise and to model a professionalism that will foster a sense of worth for the novice. In this way the art therapy supervisor remains in contact with his or her own dual inner images of self as a creator of art objects and as the artist of self-transformation.

These three primary aspects of supervision are complementary. When each is attended to properly, we begin to approach the model of supervision suggested by Greek mythology. When Odysseus prepared to leave for Troy, he entrusted the care of his household and the education of Telemachus to his faithful friend, Mentor.

The mentor model of supervision requires the establishment of an enlightened and supportive relationship in which the mentor is clearly identified as the master of the discipline. In addition to his wealth of experience and knowledge, he is dedicated to the transferring of these to the student. In the classic tradition of acceptable paradox, the mentor is above the novice in a hierarchical system, yet deeply committed to the process of the heroic journey, on which he is a fellow pilgrim. Thus the mentor is a deep resource of technical information, a participant in an institutional political system, a capable holder of the swirling emotional currents of the intern and a willing companion who will honor the quest of the student (Fig. 10).

In this age of specialization and boundary definition, the mentor traverses the blurred lines between education and therapy. The student of therapy inevitably must struggle with his or her own developmental and pathological issues that are stirred by contact with patients. The mentor's response must be to gently raise the mirror and ask the intern, "What do you see?" Learning to be an art therapist is not an exercise in memorization. There are no formulas that say, *when the patient does this, you must do that.*

Each new intern presents unique challenges to the mentor. One student may view the mentor as an unnecessary burden, an authority who must be manipulated and avoided whenever possible. Another seizes this opportunity for emotional support and subtly seeks personal therapy under the guise of instruction. Another projects unresolved parental conflicts into the relationship, setting up a battle ground in the early stages of the journey. Some see the mentor as invulnerable. Some see issues of control. Some seek protection while others long to compete. The attitude that the intern brings to the relationship has deep personal meaning.

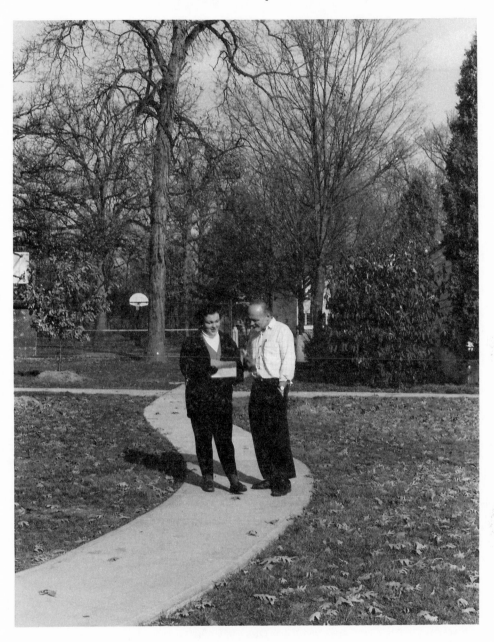

Figure 10. The mentor asks, "What do you see?"

These are the starting places for supervisor and supervisee, much like the initial transferences that the patient brings to therapy. The mentor must begin the journey by honoring the student's early feelings, in the belief that they are the first road markers. The mentor must be attentive to these early feelings, for they will give direction as to how the journey should proceed. It is the mentor's task to see the intern clearly and to approach humbly and with reverence. It is, after all, the student who is embarking on the heroic quest, the master has been this way before. The mentor must not allow any initial counter-feelings toward the intern to get in the way, but must be still and attend. While it is the student who will do most of the work, success cannot be attained without a deep and honest relationship with a supervisor.

On the students' first day in our program at Harding Hospital, I ask each one to begin keeping a journal. I ask them to write in it every day. They are to record their impressions of patients, therapists, office ambience, how they feel about being in the program, et cetera. I inform them that I will read their journals once a week, before our regularly scheduled supervisory sessions.

The journal entries of students in the first few weeks of training often bear resemblances to one another. Some questions recur:

Why am I here?
Is this what I really want to do?
How will I ever be able to understand all this?
What *is* art therapy? Is it valid?

Listen to an entry from the journal of Joan Selle:

9/12/89

Yesterday, my first day, was in some ways exciting and in other ways overwhelming. I realize how much I have to learn. By the time I arrived home yesterday I felt kind of numb. I had been bombarded by so many emotions, I hardly felt anything. Just numbness.[11]

Whether the student begins with the sense of overwhelmed numbness, or with rigidly set answers to the questions listed above, it quickly becomes evident that there are no clearcut paths to follow. The mentor patiently suggests to both the lost and the falsely secure that there are no cookbook definitions nor ready-made roles that will be enough for their journey.

In the middle of one supervisory session, my intern sat sobbing. She'd been given some critical feedback by a colleague of mine regarding her style of dress. He said it was seductive. She exclaimed, "I can't help looking the way I do. Damn it, Bruce, tell me what to do!"

I sat quietly and she continued. "If you would just give me a rule book. First I mess up in the expressive art group by not saying enough. Then I talked to a patient in the studio that I wasn't supposed to. Now *he* says I am too sexual. I give up."

I responded by telling her about Franz Kafka's character K., who so desperately wants to gain entry into THE CASTLE. K., I tell her, is anguished by the conflicting instructions he receives from the authorities of the Castle.[12] "You remind me of K.," I tell her. "You so long for someone to tell you how to go about this training program. I'm sorry, I can't do that, but I will certainly go through it with you."

Gradually the student abandons the search for pat answers and clear formulas. Some celebrate their new-found freedom to learn. Others cling stubbornly to the style of education that has become familiar to them during the first sixteen years of formal study. The transforming power of the art process eventually asserts itself and a phenomenological art therapy approach emerges. As this metamorphosis occurs, there is a coinciding decrease in the students' interest in behaviorism, coupled with an increased awareness of the existential issues faced by psychiatric patients. These changes do not happen easily. They often force an unprecedented level of anguish and introspection. At this point, the mentor must be willing to hold the pain of the apprentice.

As the interns struggle to let go of the wish for an easy way through the training process, many seek personal therapy. I see this as a strength in the novice, to search out the medicine they are prescribing to others. Now the training process becomes the acceptable paradox: supporting the student as both healer and seeker of healing.

This is a crucial experience for all involved, for it forces a new level of maturity upon the interns. They can no longer artificially separate themselves from their patients by saying, "I am here to serve you." Likewise, it thrusts upon the mentor memories of the first steps on his own journey, when he was not the master, but rather the frightened pilgrim. The intern is reminded of the common humanity of the mentor, the patient and himself. The mentor is reminded of shared experience with both patient and pupil. The patient may also feel a new sense of safety with the novice therapist.

The intern is placed in an exquisite position for learning. He must maintain a professional demeanor with the patient, even while exploring the emotional rivers within himself. Questions arise about personal integrity and honesty. How can I be of help to this patient when I feel so much turmoil myself? What good am I when I feel the same thing she does? Shouldn't I tell her the truth that I feel that way, too? Again, a passage from Joan's journal:

> Safety versus facing fear. At first I'm not sure whether this is an option or a comparison. At times I choose one, other times another. Both can be beneficial. It seems to take sensitivity and courage to make the decision. I wonder . . . can there be safety in facing your fears? I don't know.

As the interns struggle with facing their fears, they often seek the comfort of old, known intellectual territories. The student with a strong arts background suddenly expresses a new defiance towards the mentor, who is the symbol of the psychological quest. She rebels, proclaiming that she does her art for the sake of art alone. All this analysis must cease, for the preservation of her creative integrity. Students with an education or psychology background revert to old patterns of intellectualization. In either case, these theoretical retreats may be seen as defenses against the fears that emerge.

Whatever form an individual intern's resistance takes, it must be held and attended to by the mentor. For both, it is a defense against the struggle that process-oriented existential art therapy entails. The mentor must help the student integrate the polarities of art and therapy, at the same time supporting the student's personal growth.

In our clinical setting we have the advantage of having the active support of the hospital administration and the professional respect of colleagues in psychiatry, social work and psychology. The art therapists have been utilized as group leaders, co-therapists in psychotherapy groups, consultants to family therapists, adjuncts to psychotherapy and in some cases primary therapists. This is not the case in many settings, however. In some hospitals and clinics, arts therapies are viewed as little more than babysitting or leisure time management. Our students experience the pain of this sometimes subtle, sometimes overt devaluation of their chosen life's work as they venture out into satellite clinical programs.

In the past, I have felt bad about these assaults on the profession. I have longed to protect my students from such professional cruelties. I have changed my outlook on this, however. I now see that such challenges can be viewed as gifts that art therapists are given from our fellow healers. The jabs of devaluation push the intern to think clearly about what they are doing and why. We are forced to think deeply about the role the arts play in the healing of persons. As a mentor, I frame the student's painful encounter with the psychiatrist as an invaluable opportunity for the student to do one of two things: 1) the intern may be able to foster a relationship with the psychiatrist and eventually educate her or him about art therapy; 2) the intern may use the opportunity to learn about the clinic's political system. One can surely not change a system unless you know what it is.

Becoming part of an established institution such as a clinic or psychiatric hospital can be difficult for the intern whose self image is based upon personal freedom and creative expression. The struggle with, and sometimes against, the institutional system is a noble one, for it is a skirmish whose battleground is the soul. At some point each of us must come to grips with how much compromising we can do without giving up our own identity. The mentor must again hold the mirror, asking the apprentice to reflect on this aspect of the journey. At the same time, the mentor will seek his own reflection, recall his own compromises and the triumphs of his pilgrimage (Fig. 11).

The supervisor/mentors who serve the Clinical Internship in Art Therapy at Harding Hospital are expected to maintain a phenomenological approach to their students. This sort of role modeling is rather rare in institutions, yet I believe that the primary role model for a creative arts therapy student must operate from a process-oriented understanding of that role. As interns become immersed in the multiplicity of communications they receive from their patients, they are inspired and engulfed. Intrigued by the visual images, verbal offerings and myriad unspoken messages generated by the patient, the intern must have the detached support and guidance of the mentor's ego.

The apprentice art therapist is exposed to intense rage, anguish, loneliness, sexuality, the overwhelming needs of the patient. For some young students this is their first encounter with such raw power. The mentor serves as an observing ego during the dramatic first steps of the journey, filtering with the intern the multiple levels of communication. The observing ego assists the novice art therapist to take a neutral view of subjective experiences. It has been said that *being understood* by another is the grownup equivalent of being held as a small child. In this way, the observing ego (mentor) holds the intern and provides the emotional security required for the training experience.

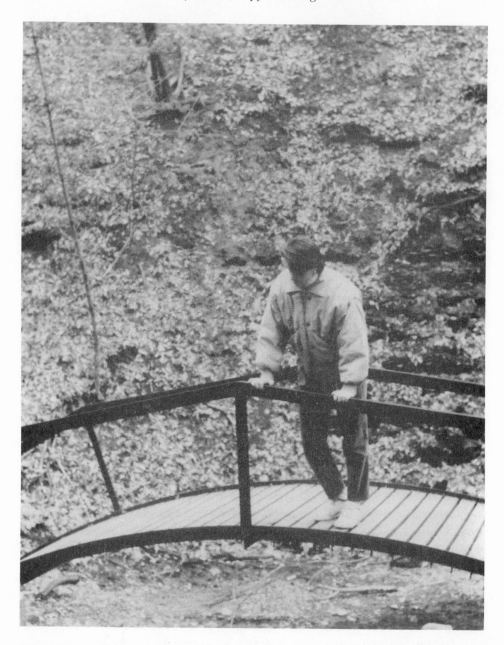

Figure 11. At some point each of us must come to grips with how much compromising we can do.

Another task of the mentor in the early phases of training is the modeling of empathy. It is from an empathic stance that the supervisor is able to console the student who has committed errors of judgment. The empathic position also allows confrontation, support and praise.

A frequent empathic confrontation has to do with the students' fantasy of themselves as healers. This naive but false self-view is very enticing. I understand their desire to regard themselves as healers. I remember my own daydreams of omnipotence. I confront these issues gently with my interns, for I have no wish to spoil their noble longings. Still, such images must be reframed as both admirable and unrealistic, and ultimately foolish. If such fantastic self-views are not reworked in the context of supervisory sessions, they will most certainly be the source of anguish for the student when he experiences his first patient suicide. Patients suffering from psychiatric illness have a variety of tragic maneuvers, all of which dramatically remind the novice and seasoned practitioner alike just who is ultimately in charge of their therapy.

The mentor stands at the side of the road in these times, softly assuring the heroic student that they have never healed anyone and never will heal anyone. The essential paradox is that the mentor longs to heal the pain of the patient and the pain of the intern, but knows that all he can do is encourage both to use the creative healing power of the art process. In such times it is most important that the supervisor engage in his own art, for if he only spoke of this to the student, who could believe him?

Not long ago one of my interns lamented, "When I see the purple scars on that young girl's arms (her patient), I ache."

I responded, "When I see you ache, I paint."

The intern grumbled, "Is that all?"

I sighed, "It has to be enough."

A central theme of art therapy training programs must be that all feelings are acceptable, whether one is a client, an intern or a therapist. We live in a culture that has separated us from the feeling process. Feelings have been categorized as "good" or "bad." Good feelings are pleasant and comfortable. Bad feelings are unpleasant and uncomfortable. Art therapists must be encouraged to abandon this hedonistic view of feelings. In our program we teach that all feelings are amoral—neither good nor bad, they simply *are.*

I try to emphasize that feelings are the tools of our trade, along with the whole range of art media. Just as no artist would condemn the use of any given medium, I encourage the intern to turn away from the cultural indoctrination that suggests that some feelings are more worthy than others.

By focusing on the acceptability of all feelings, we free the student to bring to supervision anger towards the patient, as well as pity, or disgust, or sexual attraction. Each of these *feeling responses* to patients offer growth opportunities for both the intern and the patient. Such growth would be impossible if the feelings themselves were repressed or denied.

The recurring themes of emptiness presented by borderline personality patients are particularly difficult feeling experiences for apprentices, I have found. I outlined this phenomenon in EXISTENTIAL ART THERAPY: The Canvas Mirror[3] as a pervasive experience of our time. Viktor Frankl, in MAN'S SEARCH FOR MEANING[13], describes "the existential vacuum; the vacuum being that vague sense of boredom and desolate disinterest brought about by a lack of grounding in tradition, or family spirituality. Through our mobility we have, as a people, successfully separated ourselves from our hometowns, our parents, and our extended families. We have become a culture with little or no meaningful history.

The creative art therapy student is not immune to these disturbing societal trends. The intern cannot help but identify with the themes of loneliness, anger and a history that bleed onto the canvas in the images of her patient. As an artist, she too has spent many hours of her life in isolation. She cannot help be moved by the losses depicted by her clients. Her mentor's task is to construct the boundaries she will need in her work. She must learn to separate herself from the void within her patient. She cannot allow the emptiness of another to be mistaken for her own loss. At such times the skillful supervisor will share his own struggle with detachment. The intern must experience the reality that the patient's life does not stop when the intern goes on spring vacation. I share with my students the metaphor of the guitar player.

In order to play the guitar, one must develop calluses on the fingertips. Without these, the guitarist cannot play for more than a few moments. It would simply be too painful. At the same time, the calluses must not be so thick that the sense of touch is deadened. I tell the interns, "If you really want to learn to do this work, you are going to have to learn to protect yourself."

Again the essential paradox: the therapist must always be detached enough to be able to see clearly, yet never so detached as to be out of touch with the pain of the patient. It is the same in the relationship between mentor and student. I cannot allow the intern's struggle to overwhelm me, but I must always be within easy reach.

As we journey together, student and supervisor, there is a gradual transformation taking place in the student, in me and in our relationship. Pushed by growth beyond the bounds of naivete, through the false feelings of omnipotence, the student gains a sense of self as a professional — authentic, powerful and humble before the creative healing force of the arts. The success of this endeavor weighs heavily on the shoulders of the supervisor/mentor.

While it is true that the student is the one most responsible for the outcome, the supervisor still bears the weight of being with the traveler.

This is the first of the essential elements of art therapy training.

Chapter VI

THE ART EXPERIENCE

In a videotaped interview with Don Jones, one of the American pioneers of creative arts therapy, the question was asked, "Are you an artist or a therapist?" His response was emphatic, "I am an artist." In the nearly fifteen years that I worked with Don, his answer never changed. "I AM AN ARTIST." There are no doubt others who contributed to the birth of the profession who would answer in a similar way. Today's creative arts therapists seem to lack the passion of this conviction, however. The fiery dedication to an identity as an artist has cooled.

I was teaching a course at an institute where this question became a source of controversy. I had declared that art therapists need to remain active in their own artistic media in order to preserve their authenticity as art therapists. A student who was very near graduation spoke, "Are you saying that the art therapist has to be able to paint in order to be genuine in their work?"

"No," I replied, "that's not exactly what I mean. You can paint, or sculpt, or write, or dance—whatever. The medium you choose is up to you. My point is that in order to be an art therapist, you must engage in the art process at a deep level."

The student recoiled. "No one has ever said that to me. I don't think I like this idea very much. It seems to me that it is most important that I am a good therapist who understands the theories of personality and the principles of psychotherapy. I use the art as a vehicle for relating, but I am certainly no artist in my own right."

I responded, "If the art is only an ancillary process to your therapy work, why bother calling what you do *art therapy?*"

I have had similar exchanges with my peers at both state and national art therapy conferences. It is a troublesome issue at this time within the American Art Therapy Association. It is of great concern to me that the guidelines generated by AATA for Master's Degree programs do not support continued engagement in studio art coursework. It is mentioned only in passing as a possible elective.

There is some evidence that others within the profession share this concern. My wife, Catherine Moon, ATR, and I were invited to address the annual meeting of the Art Therapy Educators Conference, on the topic, *The Art in Art Therapy.* Unfortunately we were unable to accept the invitation. It is encouraging, however, that this group, which is made up of the directors of the prominent academic programs from around the country, is concerned about these issues.

There is a longstanding sarcastic comment about educators that goes like this: those who *can,* do; those who *can't,* teach. As an art therapist, educator and artist, I respond to this notion at several levels. I believe it is essential that art therapy educators remain active in their clinical work. It is not enough to review the literature with the student. One must be able to speak from active therapeutic work. At the same time, I believe it is crucial for me as an art therapist to continue my own artistic growth and work. At still another level, I must teach in my field. It is the only way I have of repaying the mentors of my life. By remaining focused on my art, therapy and education identity, I bring honor to my teachers.

The students who come to the Clinical Internship in Art Therapy at Harding Hospital are not offered electives in studio art; they are *expected and required* to engage actively in art processes. It is not enough that they practice art as a form of parallel play in the presence of patients. They must make art that is for themselves and about themselves.

In the early days of the program, Don Jones devised a series of twenty art tasks that the intern was expected to complete during the training year. He called this *the artist's life script.* As the program has evolved over. the past decade, we have abandoned the life script format for a more open, less prescriptive studio requirement. Still a cornerstone of our program is that we regard our students as functioning artists who are in training to become therapists.

It is a mystery to me that the art process receives so little attention in academic art therapy training settings. Even more mysterious is the absence of discussion of the arts at conferences and symposia on art therapy. In all the time I have spent in lectures and meetings with fellow art therapists, I can think of only a handful of occasions when the focus of dialogue has been on the artistic endeavors of colleagues. It is almost as if we are embarrassed by our roots in the art process. I sometimes imagine peers introducing themselves as art THERAPISTS. It's not that I object to our discussions, in professional circles, of developmental theory, or transference/countertransference issues. It's just that I long for balance and creative integration.

The journey that the creative arts therapy intern makes is a complex one. It travels many paths at once. One path is littered with articles, books, lectures. One is strewn with emotional landmines, booby traps planted in the unconscious by encounters with patients. Yet another is an inward path, shaped through the integrating creative art experience. It is on this inner road that the tired and battered intern finds rest and comfort.

All students come to a crisis point in their long training journey. I suspect that all creative arts therapists experience a similar difficult period in their professional lives. The factors that precipitate are as varied as the individuals themselves. The common aspect is that when the crisis occurs, one's motivations are questioned, one's confidence is shaken and stability is disrupted. It is at this point in training and in practice that the arts processes are needed most. All too often, however, it is precisely during these periods that many students withdraw from their own art making. It is as if they believe that to engage in creative work would steal what precious energy they still possess.

Whether the crisis is brought on through the intense relating with seriously ill patients, or by the unrelenting work load of graduate school, or by personal relationships outside of the training setting, my counsel is always the same: Get back into the studio and MAKE ART.

A few years ago, a graduate of our program called me to share that he was going through a difficult time. Since leaving our program, he had gone on to be the art therapist on the psychiatric wing of a large metropolitan general hospital. After three years there, he had secured a job with a State agency and had been promoted to a high administrative post. His promotion had taken him entirely away from clinical contact with the patients the agency served. He asked if we might get together to talk things over. I suggested we meet for dinner early the next week.

As we ate he explained in detail the many changes in his life since my last contact with him. He had married, bought a house and now was the father of a son. His job paid well, almost twice what I earn in a year. Still, he was discontent. He talked for most of an hour. I listened, nodded my head, and grunted now and then. When at last he seemed to run down, I asked, "When was the last time you did any sculpture, or painted?" (One of my clearest memories of him was of his hands covered with paint.)

He sighed, "Bruce, who has the time?" For the rest of our dinner, I prodded, cajoled and coaxed him to get back to the studio.

A few months later he called me again. He said that he was quite depressed and asked if I knew anyone in private practice that I would recommend for him to go see for therapy. I gave him the name of a social worker whom I respect a great deal. As he was about to hang up, I asked, "By the way, have you done any art work lately?"

There was a long pause. "Well, I tried. Every time I started a painting, though, I couldn't stand what I was painting. It was horrible. So I quit trying."

In his most recent book, DEPTH PSYCHOLOGY OF ART[14], my friend, Shaun McNiff, says that as artists, "our purpose is one of awakening consciousness to the experience of soul."

I believe that it is impossible for art making to happen without deep psychological stirrings happening as well. This is not to say that all artists would be willing to imagine themselves as depth psychologists, nor would many have the desire to verbalize these stirrings. Still, I contend that there is soul-work taking place, consciously acknowledged or not. I think this accounts for my graduate's resistance to painting. For a variety of reasons, he did not want to be moved by his own creative forces.

The heroes of fairy-tale journeys must go through times of darkness and deep isolation. In mythology this is known as *the time of ashes,* a time of descent. The hero is helped along the way by primitive things—a stone or a wild animal. Although the hero may feel utterly lost and alone, he is eventually guided back to the light, but helped only when he most needs it.

Training to be an art therapist is a deep experience. To engage with one's art and the art of others exerts a powerful inward pull, toward the core of the self. In an era when mental health professions depend upon secular science and technology, art therapy remains a sacred pursuit. Images born during the training years, particularly in crisis periods, are manifestations of the soul-work in process. As a profession we cannot afford to stray too far from our soul—ART. I am appalled to hear my colleagues confess that they have not worked in their own media seriously since they started their forty-hour-a-week jobs, or since they got married, or since their children were born. If we abandon the art process for ourselves, we *art therapists* will eventually dry up and be blown away like dust.

As a mentor, as a peer, I insist that my students work with the stuff that is their art. I demand that they have stained hands. I urge them not to be ashamed of the paint smear on their shirts. I do this in every way I know how. I am there in the time of dark isolation. I carry a flashlight and a sketchpad. I share stories of my own journey.

When they ask me how I survived the perils of my dark caverns, I tell them the truth:

"I don't know, I guess I painted my way home" (Fig. 12).

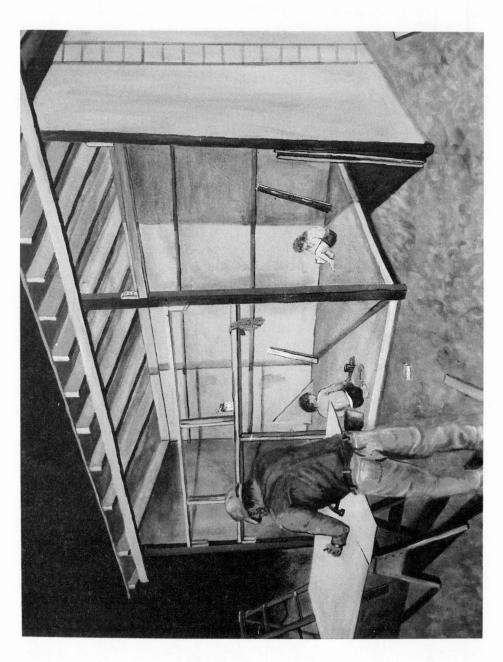

Figure 12. I guess I painted my way home.

Chapter VII

THE CORE CURRICULUM

The number of high quality art therapy training programs has expanded dramatically over the past twenty years. There has also been a substantial increase in the volume of written materials about the creative arts therapy profession. When I was a beginning student, I was frustrated that there was so little I could find to read about this new and exciting field. Today's graduate students need not feel so deprived. *The American Journal of Art Therapy, The Arts in Psychotherapy* and *The Journal of the American Art Therapy Association* have done much to disseminate articles that have deepened and enriched the fund of knowledge. Added to those publications have been the significant works of authors Shaun McNiff, Harriett Wadeson, Judith Rubin, Arthur Robbins, Myra Levick, Helen Landgarten, Janie Rhyne and others. Finally, the efforts of the American Art Therapy Association to publish and record proceedings of annual conferences has provided a wealth of information and experience that is now available to student and practitioner alike.

The availability of all this information has had a curious effect upon the professional identity of art therapists. What is most important in the training and practice of art therapy has been the subject of much debate. Shall we regard ourselves as artists first; artists who use their natural sensitivity to humanity and augment that with coursework in psychology? Or shall we describe ourselves as psychotherapists who may use the arts as an adjunct in their work with patients?

Don Jones often described himself as an artist who works with the emotionally disturbed. Harriett Wadeson states, "Art therapists should be psychotherapists plus."[15] This orientation question may seem to split semantic hairs. I believe, however, that the resolution of this question will have deep and lasting influence on the future of the profession.

Educators must decide just what we are attempting to train in the Master's program. Are we educating psychotherapists who dabble in paint or poetry, or are we shaping a profession that is unique, in which the arts are ascribed weight equal to developmental theory and abnormal psychology?

I have passionate answers to these questions. The depth and power of artistic, creative self expression impels us to a deep and broad knowledge of the arts. The art therapist must be sensitive to the pushes and pulls of *line character,* the ebb and flow of emotional currents affected by *color* and the potentialities of *weight, mass* and *emptiness* in form. Artistic sensitivities are then coupled with academic understanding of human development, psychological theory, individual, group and family dynamics, as well as systems of counseling and psychotherapy.

Educators of art therapists must resist the seduction of training their students to be as-if psychologists or pseudopsychiatrists. Programs should not train students to become marriage counselors who doodle or social workers who play with chalk, because of the political pressures generated by State licensure boards and third-party payors.

Students who want to become art therapists must insist that they be trained as art therapists and nothing less. Students who long to be verbal psychotherapists should seek the recognized routes to that end. If they want to be marital therapists, they should be encouraged to enter social work or counseling programs which emphasize marital therapy. The professional identity of the art therapist must lie in the equal weighting of both words contained in the discipline's name: ART and THERAPY.

To adopt a polarized view, whether valuing art over therapy or therapy over art, is to take a path toward weakening, if not destroying, the integrity of the art therapy profession. These elements are the *yin* and *yang* of who we are. They cannot be separated and they should not be presented in any way that devalues or over-values one from the other.

Over the past ten years, much of the discussion in the American Art Therapy Association has revolved around issues of professionalism. Many have argued that since the hierarchy of mental health professions places psychiatrists at the top, followed by psychologists and social workers, we as art therapists should do all we can to emulate these disciplines. It is my view that these arguments are based upon the false notion that professional worth is measured by the accumulation of institutional power and personal income. That kind of measurement is discomforting to me. I am unwilling to judge an art therapist's work on the basis of tax bracket or hourly fee.

Still, the lure of imitating these professions is a powerful one. We have to come to grips with the reality that our professional prestige must come from our own profession. This is not so easy. The first problem is one of definition: what exactly is an art therapist? Breaking the title down to its components is not much help. The debate over "what is art?" is centuries old. I made some attempts to describe art and art processes in my book, EXISTENTIAL ART THERAPY: THE CANVAS MIRROR,[3] but in the end I offered nothing more than elusive glimpses and wisps of mist. After years of study I still can find no definition of art that completely satisfies my quest for a description that is both simple and comprehensive. One of the best attempts I ever heard came from a patient who suggested that art is "like a window to the soul." This, however, leaves one looking for definitions of soul.

We know that the word *therapy* is derived from the Greek, *to be attentive to.* What does it mean to be attentive to the windows of the soul? We live in an age that honors science and is at best suspicious of words like *soul,* if not downright derisive.

We begin to grasp the problems of professional identity.

Science has taught people to distrust their senses. For example, the earth moves around the sun. In a non-scientific age, humans looked up at the sky and watched the sun move past them from sunrise to noon, to dusk and finally to night. Their senses told them that the sun moves. They did not feel, or see or hear the earth move. They watched the sun. What else is to be believed? The earth is still, the sun moves.

Science has taught us that it is the earth that moves and the sun is still. Science has taught us to be skeptical of what we perceive through our senses.

Our profession is integrally linked to the senses. Whether of sight or sound or touch, the arts engage the senses. There is an inherent tension between the art therapy disciplines and those with a more scientific, cognitive and empirical emphasis.

Beginning with Plato's division of the realms of mind and body, and continuing through the separation of mental/spiritual and physical in the Middle Ages, there has been a raising up of one and debasement of the other. It is as if our scientifically oriented colleagues believe that psyche can be found in the brain; that somehow it is not fused to the body. It is important to remind ourselves that the root word of *psyche* is *soul.* Where, one may ask, does the soul reside?

The problems of definition of our profession are exacerbated if and when we describe ourselves as *art psychotherapists.* One root-oriented definition might be, "one who skillfully attends to the windows of the soul." While I personally like this definition, I can easily imagine my cognitive, scientific colleagues screaming their protestations that this is no definition at all. As one psychiatrist friend of mine exclaimed, "Are you a theologian or a therapist?"

We are in a curious situation at this time regarding the mind-body split. Clearly such divisions remain in our culture. We do see evidence of some resurgence of a more unified view of humanity, however. What little there is can be attributed to the insights of psychiatry and psychotherapy. Still, the perception of a gulf between psyche and soma persists. In their text, THE EXPRESSIVE ARTS THERAPIES, Feder and Feder comment, "The relationship between mind and body is acknowledged in modern medicine, but is almost always expressed as psychosomatic, rather than somatopsychic."[16]

The arts, however, have resurfaced as a treatment for a wide variety of emotional, mental and physical disorders. Inevitably, the recognition that mind, body and spirit are interconnected has led to increased interest in the creative arts and other non-verbal therapies. There are many patients for whom traditional verbal psychiatric treatment is either inappropriate or unavailable. Ethical providers of mental health treatment are facing the reality that some people do not retain auditory stimuli; some people do not learn through dialogue; that verbalized insight is useless if not translated into meaningful action.

I think it is unfortunate that many creative arts therapy training programs have attempted to graft the arts to more established systems of educating psychotherapists. The result is a generation of art therapists who devalue themselves as professionals. They tend to mumble the *art* component of their title. This cuts them off from their own roots. It is this rootlessness that engenders collective low-esteem, and sparks debate about the "desperate need for licensure." It leads to frustration over salary, institutional power and prestige.

As educators we must return to the roots of our profession. Our task is to train professional art therapists, people who do good work for the sake of their patients' wellbeing. Our task is to lead our students on the journey to becoming "one who skillfully attends to the windows of the soul."

Core curriculum recommendations for art therapy training at the master's level state that programs "should consist of the history, theory and practice of art therapy; experience with the techniques of practice; a concern for the distinction of the appropriate therapeutic application of art therapy with different populations; psychopathology assessment and diagnosis; ethical issues and standards of practice; consideration of crosscultural mores. The core curriculum must also include supervised practical experience. A research component should be provided and opportunity for individual research projects is recommended."

The only reference to studio art is couched in condescending, negative terms. "Normally studio art courses are regarded as undergraduate prerequisites rather than sources of graduate credit." Will there be any reference at all to art processes in the guidelines for academic, institute and clinical art therapy training by the end of this decade?

One of my graduates asked me to suggest a reading list, explaining that she felt inadequate in designing art therapy exercises. "I just don't know how to think metaphorically," she said. I suggested that she read Grimm's Fairy Tales, Albert Camus's THE FALL, Melville's MOBY DICK, Robert Frost, D. H. Lawrence, Bruno Bettelheim, J. D. Salinger, W. P. Kinsella, e.e. cummings, Joseph Campbell, Robert Bly, John Donne, Kurt Vonnegut, Stephen King. . . .

My point, though exaggerated, was that literature, classic and contemporary, prose and poetry, profound and popular, is the best source of therapeutic metaphor. Literature is an interpretation of life as experienced by the artist/author. The creative arts therapist, whose task is to respond sensitively to the art (life interpretations) of the patient, needs a repertoire of literary, musical, visual and sensual memories from which to draw his response.

I am concerned that the core curriculum recommendations make no mention of these other sources of experience. We become too narrow in our thinking if our master's degree programs restrict the fields of inquiry to readings in art therapy and psychology.

An analogy may be made to the specialties in auto repair. I go to one place to have my muffler fixed, another to have the brakes adjusted. Someone else takes care of the tires and another mechanic works on engine repairs. Oil changes are done at the gas station, but when my radio quit working, it had to be sent to a service center three states away. With all that, the car still doesn't run very well and I have the uneasy feeling that no one in the world understands how an *entire* automobile functions.

The creative arts therapies are related not only to psychology and art, but to philosophy, theology, literature—all the humanities as well. All training programs should review their required courses with an eye towards studio art and these other human studies. We can train young people to attend to the windows of the soul. We must educate our students to become *masters* of creative arts therapy, not merely technicians in assessment or diagnosis.

Chapter VIII

THE CLINICAL EXPERIENCE

I do not recall exactly when I read my first description of mental illness. It might have been in high school when I discovered I NEVER PROMISED YOU A ROSE GARDEN in Senior English. Or it might have been in Psych. 101 at Bowling Green State University in Ohio. Whenever, wherever it was, I remember the sense of awe and fascination I felt as I read about schizophrenia, depression and anxiety disorders. The more I learned, the more I was captivated. I read and read and read, all the while seeking degrees in art education, theology and education, areas that had little obvious connection with mental illness.

I had heard of art therapy from my faculty advisor, Dr. Gary Barlowe of Wright State University, but I had not considered it as a possible vocation until I had entered the Methodist Theological School in Delaware, Ohio. I intended to become a pastor who specialized in counseling ministry. While in graduate school, I was hired by the Worthington Community Counseling Service, a treatment program for adolescents. My job description was not very specific. Somehow I was to relate to troubled teenagers through music and the visual arts, provide evening and weekend telephone counseling, drop-in crisis intervention and suicide hotline counseling.

With the innocent courage of the young I was confident that all of my reading and coursework had prepared me well for this position. I was sure that I was equal to the task. I would not disappoint the center's director, Kent Beittel. Since Kent had faith in me, I was secure, though a novice.

My first client appeared on my second night on duty. She was not an adolescent, but she was quite troubled. Her hair was a wild, uncombed tangle. She smelled of days without a bath. Her eyes darted around the office. When I asked her to sit down, she recoiled, flattening her body against the door.

Client: No, my God, no! Do you think I am just going to walk in here and do anything you want me to?

Bruce: Well, of course not. I just thought you'd be more comfortable sitting down. Can I be of help?

Client: You can make them leave me alone.

Bruce: Who are you talking about?

Client: The thugs at the halfway house.

She lit a cigarette and began to circle the room. My mind raced, filled with anxiety:

This woman is scary. She's not supposed to be here. I'm only supposed to talk with kids. What halfway house? What thugs? What's she going to do with me? I wish she'd sit down. Why am I here alone? I should have taken that teaching job. My God, what do I do?

Eventually the woman did calm down. She was able to telephone the psychiatric halfway house where she was a resident. They sent a staff member over to pick her up and return her to the house. Later I learned that she was a chronic paranoid schizophrenic who had episodes like this every now and then. She had been to most of the community counseling centers in the city at one time or another.

This information was of little use to me. I was angry with myself because I had panicked. I had been unable to think clearly and had not had a clue as to how best to help the woman, even though her behavior was straight out of the textbook. That was when I learned that *reading* about a psychiatric disorder is very different from being in the presence of a human being who *has* that disorder.

This incident, illuminating the difference between the clinical description and living reality, illustrates why clinical experience is essential for the art therapy student. The recommendations of the American Art Therapy Association for art therapy training leading to a Master's degree are:

Art Therapy Experience

Opportunities should be provided for students to undergo the direct experience of the therapeutic process, as a means toward both personal growth and the development of skills needed by art therapists. Encouragement should be given to students who wish to engage in more extensive self-explorations; however, a clear distinction between teaching and therapy should be maintained. Students desiring personal therapy should engage therapists who have no teaching, supervisory or administrative responsibility within the training program.

Practical Training Opportunities

Training in the field is discussed under two headings: field work and practicum (sometimes called internship).

1) **Field Work.** It is strongly urged that classroom instruction be enriched by field work. Approaches and ideas discussed in the classroom should be tested in practice, from the beginning stages of the program. The academic and clinical studies should be closely coordinated throughout the two years of training. Field work preceding or following the practicum in the same setting is often valuable for the sake of more sustained experience. To provide contact with a broad variety of clients, total field experience should usually take place in several different settings. The number of hours to be spent in field work may be more flexibly determined than practicum hours.

2) **Practicum.** A minimum of 600 hours of supervised art therapy experience is required, half of which must include group, family and/or individual client contact using art therapy. The remaining hours include related activities such as conferences with supervisors, case review, record keeping and participation in staff meetings.[17]

These official AATA statements send a double message. At first glance they appear to "strongly" urge programs to structure meaningful clinical experience as a component of the educational program. However, looking deeper, these statements are disturbing. I am particularly uneasy about the 600 hours of supervised art therapy experience. When 600 hours are spread over a two-year period, it averages out to roughly two hours a day. Presumably half of those two hours will be spent in "related activities," leaving only one hour per day being spent with patients doing art therapy. In such a practicum there is little opportunity for a consistent, integrated experience for the student. It might be even worse to have the student at a practicum site for only two days a week, but for more hours each day. If that were the case, the student would be able to get a better feel for the flow of a given day, but would have no opportunity to experience the flow of a week, or a month, at the site.

Healthcare institutions have a life and rhythm of their own. Students need to learn how to be a part of the system. It cannot be done by being at the site for only two hours a day or two days a week. In order to learn the life-system of the institution, the student must have a significant period of time to work consistently within the system. Creative arts therapy must be taught in the context of practical reality. Therefore, I suggest that the AATA recommendations regarding field work should be altered to read, "It is strongly urged that clinical field work experiences be enriched by classroom instruction."

It is essential that creative arts therapy students learn the role their discipline plays in the treatment milieu. To do this, they must also understand the roles of social workers, psychiatrists, psychologists, nurses, attendants, childcare workers, maintenance personnel, administrators, chart reviewers, recreation therapists, pharmacists and horticulture therapists, not to mention unit rules and hospital policies. Only when one understands all of these components can one understand and articulate one's own unique contribution to the patient. There is simply no way this can be done in brief, inconsistent clinical exposures.

Chapter IX

SCIENCE AND SOUL IN THE CLINICAL SETTING

Clinical treatment settings in the 1990's are undergoing massive changes in response to the demands of health maintenance organizations, third party payors and increased competition. Advances made in bio-neurological understandings and treatment of mental disorders will also affect the nature of care provided in clinical settings. Already at the time of this writing, the average length of stay in inpatient psychiatric hospitals, both private and state run, have dropped dramatically over the past few years. The language of treaters has shifted from the poetic, abstract and qualitative regarding patient care toward the functional, concrete and quantifiable.

In *Existential Art Therapy: The Canvas Mirror,* I stated my firm belief that what we do as creative arts therapists cannot be measured.[3] My friend and colleague, Shaun McNiff, asserts that we must reclaim our roots in a view of the arts as an "unconscious religion,"[14] and turn with all due respect away from over-scientification of our field. Another colleague, Sr. Kathleen Burke of Ursuline College, has expressed concern over the increasing popularity of assessment procedures used by arts therapists. Her concern is that it reflects an attempt to concretize and quantify arts phenomena.

We are not alone in this identity struggle. Similar concerns are raised by psychiatrists, social workers, recreation therapists and even, on occasion, clinical psychologists. Speaking most clearly about this dilemma is the noted psychologist and prolific author, James Hillman. In the first pages of his work, *Re-Visioning Psychology,* he writes, "This book is about soul making. It is an attempt at a psychology of soul, an essay in re-visioning psychology from the point of view of soul. This book is therefore old-fashioned and radically novel because it harks back to the classical notions of soul and yet advances ideas that current psychology has not even begun to consider."[18]

Professionals at all levels within clinical settings are experiencing an identity crisis and a crisis of conscience. We have been forced to examine

65

critically who we are and what we do in the service of our patients and clients. Our sense of integrity has been battered by the reality of a severely limiting financial system in which the determinant of care given is almost never the needs of the patient, and almost always the whim of faceless insurance reviewers. The well insured or individually wealthy receive appropriate treatment while the rest are allocated emotional band-aids.

Still, the clinical setting is the essential locale for meaningful training in the creative arts therapies. Therefore, it is imperative that attention is given the student in relation to this continuum of science and soul. Not only do educators have a responsibility to the student in this regard, but the student has an important role as well. The student's task is to question what *is*. The question may spark a dialogue that can rekindle one's courage in the face of systems wrestling with their own soul.

To understand my wariness about the scientification of the helping professions in general and the creative arts therapies in particular, consider the comments of Freud on the development of psychoanalysis. He pointed out " . . . what it began working upon was the symptom, a thing that is more foreign to the ego than anything in the mind." I fear that by attempting to align our teaching of art processes too closely to the methods of science, we run the risk of pathologizing the arts. Any sensible art therapist knows the damage that superficial psychological inquiries can have on the works of artists. Such tactics have been employed by some authors on the lives of Van Gogh, Picasso, Pollack and others, thus giving the public the misguided notion that the arts are the realm of madmen.

On the other hand, if arts therapies in the clinical training setting are approached from a perspective of *soul*, the work becomes sacred. While I embrace the concept that art comes from the depth of human beings, out of turmoil and conflict and passion, I believe it to be a healthy process, not a pathological ventilation.

Having said this, I feel compelled to assure the reader that I am not really anti-science, especially when science is related to human well-being. Who can question the near-miraculous benefit of lithium to persons suffering from bi-polar disorder? Who doubts the positive contributions of bio-neurology in the treatment of schizophrenia? My point is not to devalue science, but to bring honor to the intuitive, soul-making processes of the arts.

By suggesting that arts-making is soul-making, I mean that art processes offer a new perspective. Painting, dancing and writing makes meaning possible by turning random events into meaningful experiences. I suggest that there is an artistic foundation to human existence and a perspective that cannot be pinpointed as the property of behavior or language or society or brain physiology. The special gift of the creative arts therapies to the patient and to the clinical setting is this soul/art-making process. It is the work that only we can do.

It is essential that educational programs in the creative arts therapy disciplines impart not only the mechanics of the profession, but the philosophical underpinnings as well. When this is done, the student is prepared to understand not only the treatment of individuals and groups, but the functions of systems, hierarchy and political issues that are integral within mental health institutions.

Chapter X

THE WORK OF ART THERAPY

Ms. Lou Powers, whom you met earlier in this book, is a graduate of the Clinical Internship in Art Therapy at Harding Hospital. She recently completed her academic work toward the Masters of Art in Expressive Therapy at Lesley College, Cambridge, Massachusetts. Shortly after she returned from a five-week summer intensive at the Lesley campus, she shared with me the joy of the relationships she had made there and the relief and satisfaction that accompanied the completion and acceptance of her thesis. Lou's face glowed as she told me of her friends and experiences in the Boston area. I commented, "It sounds like a wonderful time, Lou. It must have been fun."

Her expression changed immediately. She said, "It was very hard work." An awkward silence hung between us briefly.

The intensity of this sudden shift in emotional tone in our conversation heightened my awareness of just how hard the work is, for students, teachers and therapists alike.

Webster's defines work as "physical or mental effort exerted to do or make something; purposeful activity, labor, toil . . . to strain . . . to cause or bring about . . . to cultivate, to cause to function . . . to ferment . . . "[10]

The work of learning to be, being and teaching about being an arts therapist is strenuous, straining, purposeful, toil. It is not easy.

In his conversations with Bill Moyers titled, *The Power of Myth,* Joseph Campbell gives the image of the warrior: one who is able to discipline their efforts and "follow their bliss."[19] By his own description, Campbell lived the warrior role as he disciplined his inquiry into the myths of various cultures, at times reading eight to ten hours a day. This is passionate discipline.

Perhaps passionate discipline is an apt description of the work involved in becoming an art therapist. Here again a reference to the artistic process is relevant. The products of our artistic endeavors are described as *art works,* or *works of art.* No one would dare to look at the Sistine Chapel and marvel over Michaelangelo's *avocational* pursuits. It is his *work!* As fanciful and playful as Calder's mobiles may appear, few would question the work they required.

Reviewing the work of any artist, one comes to grips with the sum of his or her effort, strain and purposeful toil; the ability to be patient and passionate as the work proceeds through the artist's personal history. One finds measures of willingness to tolerate internal storms and fermentations; traces and hints of the physical effort demanded by the art. The work of the artist is not easy, covered with blisters, both physical and emotional, tired muscles, cramped fingers and weary eyes. The life's work of an artist is a testament to faith that the struggle was worth it, that it mattered.

Such "mattering" must lie at the core of the student, practitioner and teacher. This profession demands passionate discipline and faith in the struggle. Judy Rubin comments on this aspect of the work in *The Art of Art Therapy:*

"... It is possible to master the art of many things, such as piano playing, gourmet cooking, crewel embroidery and to do them well ... but to do them in such a way that people sigh when they hear one's sonatas, or eat one's mousse, or view one's wall hangings requires something above and beyond the mastery of the art form itself—something best identified as artistry."[20] What Ms. Rubin calls artistry, I would describe as passionate discipline.

The misinformed may speak of works of art as the product of genius or talent. While certainly gifts and talent may have a role in the development of artistry, I would recall Lou Powers's statement, "It was very hard work." No artist can rely solely upon genius to produce. The artist must do the work.

So it is with arts therapists. There are surely some students who bring to the training experience a certain wholesome, healthy, warmth that is intrinsically charismatic. These inherent characteristics alone are not enough to produce an arts therapist. Nor is intellectual capacity enough, nor artistic sensibility, nor concern for humankind. None of these attributes are sufficient in isolation. The would-be art therapist must bring a passionate discipline that will patiently blend the charisma, warmth, artistic perspective and skill, love for humanity and intellect with a willingness to work.

In the transition from undergraduate to graduate work, an intriguing transformation should occur in the student. In undergraduate school, there are inevitably courses and assignments that one must do in order to proceed. These are in some measure, hoops to be jumped through. The student recognizes them when they come up. Such hoops inspire less than excellent work. In fact, they encourage half-hearted efforts to get by and move on.

Graduate school, however, presents the student with an environment that is (or ought to be) dedicated to the individual student's personal investment in his or her own excellence. Graduate school should mark the end of academic hoop-jumping. In our program, as is the case in most settings, I am sure, there can be no room for slipshod, half-hearted effort. The students must transform their sense of identity as the hoop-jumping slave of a faculty to a new, mature view of self as a dedicated colleague of master practitioners. This is not an easy transition to make, but the work of training demands it.

In an interview published by Giovanni Papini in 1934, Sigmund Freud is quoted, "Everybody thinks that I stand by the scientific character of my work and that my principal scope lies in curing mental maladies. This is a terrible error that has prevailed for years and that I have been unable to set right. I am a scientist by necessity and not by vocation. I am really by nature an artist . . . and of this there lies an irrefutable proof: which is that in all countries into which psychoanalysis has penetrated it has been better understood and applied by writers and artists than by doctors."[21]

Our history as artists-therapists is suggested in this interview. It seems apparent that Freud understood the central role that creativity and imagery played in his infant field of inquiry, psychoanalysis.

The graduate student must be welcomed into the transformational process, and honored as one who is endeavoring to follow a rich tradition. This suggests an attitude of reverence on the part of the instructor/mentor toward the student. Such an attitude is the marker for the student that the transformation has begun. To be held in high regard by one's mentor is often a new experience for the student, but it is crucial for both parties. For the student it is, in a sense, an initiation, a welcoming to the professional realm. For the mentor/instructor or supervisor it is a reminder of the seriousness of the task. By revering the student, they guard against routinized interactions. Such an attitude by no means insures quality instruction, but it may increase the likelihood of success for the student.

The three threads of emphasis in this book—student, educator, practicing art therapist—are tightly interwoven in the fabric of our profession. It is absolutely clear to me that in order to do effective art therapy one must possess passionate discipline. It is this quality that enables one to avoid the boredom of routine involvement. Whether in the role of teacher or student, supervisor or therapist, there can be no boredom if one stays in contact with the creative challenge of the work.

Each new student offers the teacher/supervisor myriad possibilities and obstacles. Each new patient brings the therapist a mystery longing to be understood. Each new book, article, class or instruction presents the student with an invaluable opportunity to explore. This is the work that we do.

The patient's ability to make the therapeutic journey is directly correlated with the passionate discipline of the therapist. (I suggest that this applies to all therapeutic disciplines.) The art therapist's passionate discipline is likewise proportionate to that of his or her teachers, mentors and supervisors.

I close this chapter with a call to all in the field: *Attend to your passions.* If you have lost the zeal that once powered your journey, return to the studio, for it is there that you first stumbled upon the power of images and art processes. It is there that you must return when passions have cooled or discipline dissolved.

As I paint, I rediscover the work. I experience the struggle, the confusion, the painful artistic frustrations. It reminds me of my student years. It recalls the faces of patients I have known, and I hear the voices and questions of my students.

What does all this mean?

What does all this mean?

This is the work of art therapy (Fig. 13).

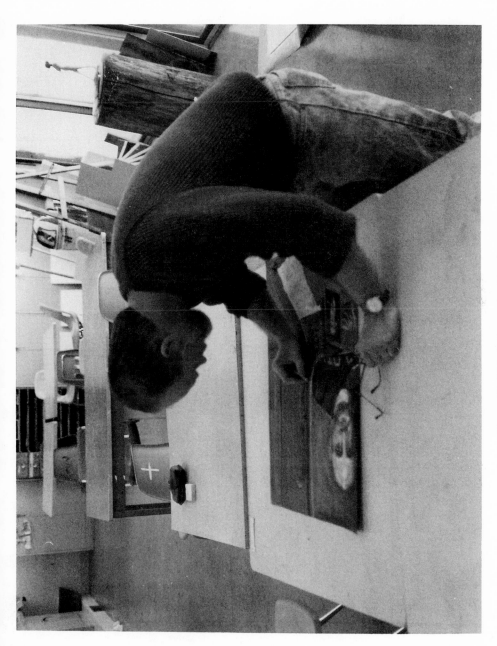

Figure 13. This is the work of art therapy.

Chapter XI

GIFTS OF THE YOUNG

*It went zip when it moved and bop when
it stopped Brrr when it stood still I never
knew just what it was and I guess I never
will.*

Tom Paxton, *The Marvelous Toy*[22]

Journal Entry:

Yesterday, my first day, was in some ways exciting and in other ways overwhelming. I realize how much I have to learn. By the time I arrived home last night I felt kind of numb. I had been bombarded by so many emotions I hardly felt anything. Just numbness. Then there are all the weird feelings of being the new kid on the block. Trying to come into a space that is new, not your own and full of a zillion things that have been happening that you have no clue about.

This morning as I listened to the reports about different patients and observed the people in the office, I wondered if they had some dichotomy between their personal and professional lives. I heard people talk about sharing feelings, being open and honest, developing good communication skills, etc., but were these things a part of their private lives? I don't know. I hope that I can learn, for myself and others too . . . I have a lot of abbreviations to learn. I think I'll write down all the ones I don't know this afternoon at the meeting and then ask some people what they are.

September, 1989
Joan Selle

Becoming an art therapist is not an easy task. The doing of therapy demands a level of maturity and self acceptance that is rare in the graduate student. It isn't their fault. In all likelihood it isn't anyone's fault. It's just the way things are.

In the summer of 1990 my wife Cathy and I went to a Tom Paxton concert in Columbus, Ohio. I was fascinated as I watched this well-known folk singer, who had recorded several albums and written countless songs that I love, interact with the children in the audience. The concert was held outside in a park. The stage was set on top of a rise in the ground. Little kids ran up the hill, unimpressed by his list of musical accomplishments and unaware of the social conventions forbidding approaching a star. Their interest was in rolling down the hill, giggling and wrestling with one another. I paid close attention, since my own kids were part of the chaos in front of Tom Paxton. I began to be embarrassed by their antics until I noticed the pleasure on the singer's face as he watched the rolling, tumbling, joyful scene before him. For a while he gave up singing his protest songs and social-consciousness ballads. Instead he offered *The Marvelous Toy, My Favorite Game* and several other ditties suited to the children. He was neither offended nor distracted by the kids' engagement in life, but seemed to feed on their energy.

When a new intern or a new class of students enter the training process, it is easy for the seasoned professional to become irritable at their naivete, their innocence, their wide-eyed questioning about why things are the way they are. It is not unusual for graduate students to enter art therapy training programs directly after completion of their undergraduate degrees. Generally such students have not yet been married, had children, suffered divorce or lost loved ones through death. Vestiges of the adolescent's sense of immortality and idealism are blended with powerful sexual drives and a deep yearning for a solidified sense of who they are. They bring energy, enthusiasm and willingness to challenge the status quo. Many bring a lively and healthy curiosity, an interest in soul-searching and introspection, but this is not always the case. Recent undergraduates have been in a nearly constant state of transition for the past ten years of life. They have gone from childhood through the rigors of adolescence and now find themselves on the front edge of responsible adulthood. In the best of circumstances, it has been a tough decade.

Now they enter the world of graduate study to become therapists. There will be reading, papers and academic hoops to jump through. They will also be required to do self-exploration, self-challenge and honest self-evaluation. For many students it is contrary to all of their personal experience.

I am reminded continually by my students that things that are routine and commonplace for me (for instance, doing a drawing with my patients about a *need* that I have) are intensely threatening to the student's sense of privacy. While students must confront and learn to deal with such things, I must also remember to honor how hard this may be for them.

The graduate student may experience profound discomfort when joining an already-established arts psychotherapy group. While the other members of the group have had time to get to know one another, the student is introduced cold to the situation. If the group cultural norm is one of self-revelation and intimacy, the student may feel extreme internal pressure to conform. The result can be a disorienting sense of inadequacy, which most often is expressed through devaluing or anger toward the program or supervising ATR. It is essential that art therapy educators and supervisors respond with empathy to students' fears and pressures.

As Joan Selle recorded in her journal, the student is made aware quickly of how much there is to learn. It can be an overwhelming realization, and unless it is appropriately addressed it can lead to destructive, self-defeating acting out by the student.

It may also be helpful, particularly for the younger student in the first stages of the educational journey, to suggest the additional support of individual therapy. The student will be exposed to forces that it is likely they have never encountered. Focus on unconscious motivations of others, horrific patient histories, mingled with intense daily interactions, pushes the student hard for personal growth and deepening. In the Harding Hospital program, supervisors regularly remind the interns that these fifteen months of training may be some of the most difficult they will ever experience. The time can also be exciting, even fun, but personal therapy may be beneficial to their professional growth. I have often been aware, as a primary supervisor, that student material brought to the supervisory session would be better handled in a more contained, exclusive session.

There are three areas that have the most potential for problems for the younger student in the training environment. First is the struggle to define oneself as an adult. If the student has gone directly from high school to undergraduate school and then to graduate study in arts psychotherapy, there has been little opportunity to function as an independent adult. This young person is quickly placed in therapy situations, often with patients much older than the student. The internal refrain is, " . . . how can I be therapeutic for this 40-year-old businessman . . . what do I know about the pressures and stress he has endured that led him to his depression?" These are valid and serious concerns for the intern and must be addressed by the teacher/supervisor.

I remember how inept I felt as a 52-year-old man wept in an art therapy session, sharing feelings about his impotence. What did I know of his experience? I was 23 years old. Oh, I knew what the word impotence meant, but the reality was so far removed from my experience that I was in no way able to be genuinely empathetic. Similarly, one of my interns approached me with her discomfort about her inability to respond to a woman suffering post-partum depression. Although the intern had researched the topic, she was still unable to grasp the depth of the mother's experience.

It is not a crime to be young, but we educators must be sensitive to our students' inadequacies based upon their lack of experience. It is best for the supervisor to be looking for gaps in the student's knowledge and experience, and to have prepared an empathetic yet reality-based response.

Second, beyond developmental problems, there is the student's struggle to form a professional identity. It is not an easy transition to make from undergraduate to art therapist-in-training. Focus must be shifted away from concern with grade point averages, a sense that school is a series of vaguely relevant hoops to be jumped through; toward a focus on the learning process as being integrally tied to the lives of others, i.e., future patients. This is a radical shift. To some degree also, students must get the message that the life of a healer is not simply an 8:00 to 5:00 occupation, but rather an approach to life. Being a therapist is a little like being a physician or a minister—you are IT all the time.

Several years ago, one of my interns learned a painful lesson. She attended a party given by one of her old college friends. In the midst of the party she was approached by a former patient who had also been invited by a mutual acquaintance. They ended up sharing jokes with each other about various hospital staff, routines, and so forth. In this social situation, the intern said some things that were inappropriate but would probably have been harmless had not the former patient been readmitted to the hospital a few weeks later. Their encounter eventually came to light in an expressive art therapy group. The intern had to be removed from participation in the group. She was deeply embarrassed and it took quite some time to undo the damage to her self-esteem that the incident had caused.

A related issue is confidentiality. It is hard for some students to adhere to this requirement, but it is essential. When I was an intern, one of my patients was part of a family that were friends of my sister and her husband. It was very difficult to deflect my sister's questions about the patient.

Another serious matter is that of receiving gifts from patients. The young student often longs to be thought of as significant or important by the patient. We struggle with this issue every Christmas. Invariably a patient purchases a gift for one of my students as a way to say, "thank you for all you are doing." I tell the student that it is inappropriate to accept such a gift. It is painful for the intern to refuse, yet to accept it would be to change the nature of the relationship from therapeutic to that of friends.

One of my students entered a supervisory session appalled at a statement my colleague, Deb DeBrular, had made to a patient. During a group feedback exercise, the patient had said to Deb, "I think you are one of the best friends I've ever had." Deb's response was, "That's nice, but you need to know that I am not your friend." The intern was angry at Deb for being so harsh and unfeeling. The task of the supervisory session became one of reframing for the student the nature of patient/therapist relationships. It became an invaluable experience for the student as she wrestled with her own wishes to be accepted and liked by patients. It gave us an opportunity to work on the student's own evolving professional identity.

A third area of difficulty for all students, but particularly for the younger student, is the process of exposing their vulnerabilities to patients by engaging in their own art work in the studio and in groups. This is an area of controversy within the profession at large. Some argue that the therapist should never draw or paint in the presence of the patient. I take exception. I believe that such concerns are the outgrowth of misguided attempts to operate from a neo-Freudian position of blank-screen neutrality. Art therapists should not pretend to be analysts. The art process calls for engagement, not false detachment. If the art therapist does not draw or paint, the range of response to the patient is unnecessarily limited to the verbal. This is an illogical paradox without validity.

Even so, it is evident that the therapist must pay attention to *what* and *when* to share through personal art making. I believe that our own words should be used only to verify the messages of the graphic images the patient creates. That is to say I think the communications of real consequence are meta-verbal. The same is true of therapist/trainee images. Students must be sensitive to what they are communicating to the patient through the images they share.

As an intern, Joan Selle was part of a girls' expressive group co-lead by Lori Brown, R. N., and me. Just before one group meeting, Joan and I had been in a supervisory session. She had become angry with me, but we had not had time to bring our conflict to resolution. The task of the group that day was to portray a feeling that you had been struggling with. Joan thought it would be inappropriate to share her anger with me in the group, so she chose to do a drawing on the theme of emptiness. In fact, she decided to leave her paper blank, thinking that the vacant brown page was enough.

As others in the group worked on their drawings, I sensed Joan's anger and resistance. I insisted that she draw something. She glared at me, then proceeded to cover her entire paper with light brown, almost the same color as the paper. As members of the group shared their work, Joan remained silent. At one point, one of the adolescent girls said, "There's something weird in this group today." The patient had picked up on the unspoken anger that had been passively expressed on Joan's "empty" page.

For several months following this event, whenever Joan and I met for supervision, I would begin the session with, "Well, Joan, let's talk about that day when you did not want to draw in expressive group." This set the stage for meaningful dialogue between us, revolving around issues of resistance, authority conflict and professional identity. It was no coincidence that during this same period, in the expressive therapy group there were recurrent themes related to trust, vulnerability and the expression of anger between adolescents and adults.

The struggles of the educational journey for younger students go hand in hand with the joys. These students often bring a level of enthusiasm, energy and commitment that outweighs their naivete and lack of experience and enables them to leap over the developmental hurdles.

As an educator and mentor, I am grateful for the novice. They rekindle in me some of the wonder and awe at the power of art and the process of therapy. I recapture some of the way I felt after my first art psychotherapy group. Through the interns' wrestlings, I experience again the pain of my first disappointments and failures. Briefly, I revisit the old anger at institutional systems that often serve themselves more than the patient. I am a comrade with my students as they run their idealistic heads into the walls of bureaucratic tradition.

Each time a new intern enters training, I remind myself that these are priceless gifts the student offers; a steady transfusion of life blood to the profession.

Chapter XII

GIFTS OF THE MALE AND FEMALE STUDENT

In November, 1988 I participated in a weekend Tavistock group relations training experience conducted by the A. K. Rice Institute in
Cincinnati. The Tavistock model is an intense, pressurized experience.
I sat with a colleague and friend, waiting for the first session to start. He
commented on the sexual makeup of the group. There were roughly
seventy trainees, of whom five were men and sixty-five were women. He
expressed some surprise and discomfort that we were so clearly in the
minority. I don't recall exactly how I responded, but I do remember
thinking, "So what else is new?"

As a male art therapist I have been in the minority in my profession
for the past seventeen years. I remember feeling a little like my colleague,
Jeff, back in 1975 when I attended a meeting of the American Art
Therapy Association for the first time. Before that conference, every
art therapist I had met was a man. My mentor was Don Jones, and many
of the stories I had heard were about men in the field. As I approached
the registration desk of the Galt Hotel in Louisville, Kentucky, I was
amazed to see so many women and so few men. If I had to guess I would
estimate that no more than five percent of the art therapists in the
United States are male.

The dynamic that emerged in the Tavistock weekend revolved around
gender/political/power issues and sexual issues. The males came to be
regarded as the precious resource. I would argue that the same is true
within the art therapy profession. This is not to devalue the significant
contributions of women to our field, but rather to acknowledge the need
of our discipline for balance.

The need for balance suggests a parallel need for an awareness of and
sensitivity to the special needs of male art therapists in training. To
understand the peculiar predicament of men in the profession, it will be
helpful to explore the developmental differences between men and women.

For several years I had the opportunity and pleasure to work as
co-therapist with Debra DeBrular in expressive arts psychotherapy groups.

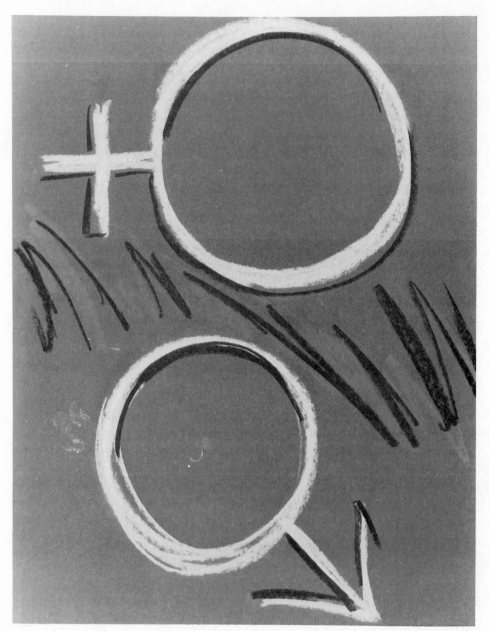

Figure 14. The differences are as powerful and deep as one can imagine.

One group was made up of six severely disturbed adolescent boys, aged 15 to 17. The group was an excellent place to explore our differences as Deb and I approached the task of treating these difficult and resistive patients.

One day we introduced a symbolic group feedback exercise. Each member had drawn from a hat the name of another. Their task was to portray the person whose name they had drawn as some kind of plant, an animal and a machine. Deb speaks:

"I'm always interested in how a patient will portray me. I surveyed the completed drawings, wondering who had chosen my name. My eyes fell on a drawing of a rose, a rabbit and an oven.

"Oh, I thought, that one is me.

"Now, in no way do I see myself as being like a rabbit, a rose, or an oven. No ... I would portray myself as perhaps like a gull, hunting above the sea, making nourishment of both the fresh fish and the garbage. Or like the hearty forsythia that blooms against the odds of the cold in the early spring. And comparing myself to a machine, I'd be an industrial sewing machine, rugged and sewing strong bonds.

"Still, I selected this picture of a rabbit, a rose and an oven as symbolic as myself. I was, after all, the only female member of that group. The other papers contained images of grizzly bears, army tanks, falcons, etc. Easily, no boy had characterized me in that way. I had been symbolized not as the flesh and blood person who lives in these clothes, but as the skirt.

"As Peter, the boy who had drawn the picture, explained his drawing to me, he said he saw me as warm, soft and pretty. I was unable to suppress my giggle at the irony of the situation. He had passed me by as a person, but still I believe he meant his portrayal of me as a compliment. While I might have preferred a more gutsy image of myself, I didn't really mind being thought of as warm or pretty.

"Aware of my thoughts and sharing a bit of my laughter, Bruce intervened, bringing to the group's collective mind a more realistic view of me. Ovens can burn, he said. And adding a bit of drama, he acted out for them how he had been pricked by my thorns. Even Bruce didn't dare comment on the potential symbolism of the rabbit."[23]

Through many such encounters with sexual stereotyping and gender-based developmental differences, I began to be more sensitive to the unique patterns and metaphors of growth that my maleness has fostered. The differences are as powerful and deep as one can imagine. For far too long they have been the basis for conflict between women and men over power and prestige. We must begin to address them not as battlefields but as potential gifts that we men and women arts therapists have to offer one another.

To begin looking at some traditional themes in masculine development, I will share with you a brief passage from Allan Sillitoe's *The Loneliness of the Long Distance Runner.*

"All I knew was that you had to run, run, run, without knowing why you were running, but on you went, through fields that you didn't understand and into woods that made you afraid, over hills without knowing you'd been up and down, and shooting across streams that would have cut the heart out of you had you fallen into them. And the winning post was no end to it, even though the crowds might be cheering you in, because on you had to go."[24]

In Sillitoe's portrait of the runner we are presented with an image of loneliness, strenuous performance, competition and unclarity about the point of it all. These are poignant themes that men confront daily in their lives. From early childhood we are taught the worth of individual accomplishment, mastery and the joy of beating your opponent.

In the years that I worked in co-therapy with Deb and in my marriage as well, I have spent much energy trying to understand my developmental experience. In doing so, I have come to grips with what I bring to a group, to co-therapy relationships and to teaching encounters with predominantly female students.

In an article titled *Male Sexuality and Masculine Spirituality* [25], Dr. James B. Nelson draws profound parallels between the masculine body and the recurrent themes it generates. " . . . without intending a biological determinism, we can still acknowledge that the male biological experience encourages certain tendencies different from those commonly experienced by women . . . "

Nelson goes on to delineate some of the body metaphors. "Male genitals are external, visible and easily accessible to touch . . . generating a greater tendency to focus and reinforce male sexual feelings in the genitals. Also, particularly in adolescence, the male experiences erections at awkward times and in unwanted situations, an experience which tends to persuade him that the penis is beyond voluntary control."

From my own experience I can echo this sentiment. I can clearly remember having to carry my three-ring notebook discreetly placed over my midsection in order to retrieve papers from my English teacher's desk in the eighth grade. It was almost as if my penis planned to embarrass me daily.

A further validation of this mind-of-its-own phenomenon is the tendency of many men to give their penis a name other than their own name. This supports the notion that it has a life and will separate from the rest of the body. This leads to the male perspective that sexual experience is focused in an act in which they must perform.

Women tend to experience their sexuality as a mysterious internal process, while a man experiences his sexual body as an implement or tool designed to explore or penetrate the feminine mystery.

Nelson goes on, "All these bodily experiences appear to incline men toward certain spiritual contours. One is externality. Mystery is less within than out there. Mystery is to be penetrated by a self which is demarked by specific boundaries." Here again we glimpse the masculine accent upon act and performance as opposed to relationship and meaning.

When I was four or five years old I was given a basketball for my birthday. A bushel basket was nailed to a door in our basement. I quickly learned that there was much praise and recognition to be gathered by my hours of practicing alone. I was a very good boy when I learned to dribble with both hands. I recall few such rewards for my developing relating skills. By the time I was seven I was sure that a man had to do the important things by himself, and that if I practiced I could learn to perform the actions skillfully (Fig. 15).

Another body metaphor stems from the physical position of the testicles. This most vulnerable part of the male body is hidden away, tucked behind the penis and between the legs. Perhaps the bio-metaphor is *protect your vulnerability, keep it secret.* This is paradoxical, of course. In order for the testicles to do what they are designed to do, i.e., make sperm, they must hang loose, away from the body, in order to maintain the correct temperature. The paradox is that while you must protect and hide your vulnerability, if you want to participate in the most profoundly intimate creative act, *you must be vulnerable.*

In addition, the musculature of the male lends itself to visions of domination, overpowering and defeat of the other. These images give insight of the roots of the difficulties men often have with intimacy. For many men there is comfort in expression of the competitive drive, discomfort in being close to someone else. In myriad social encounters during their early years, men are presented with the messages: big boys don't cry; there's nothing to be afraid of; you have to take care of things

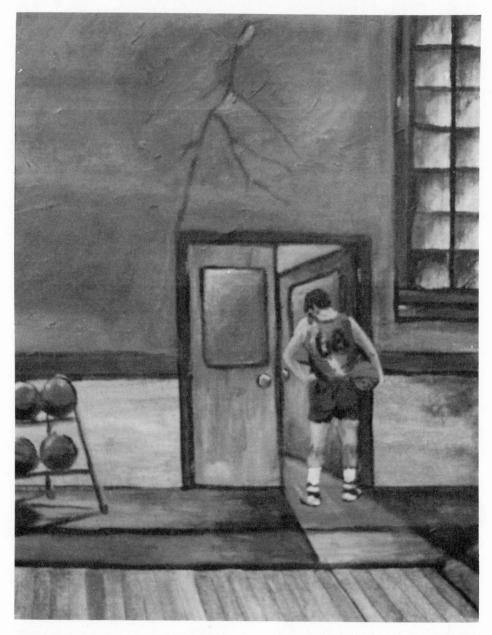

Figure 15. By the time I was seven I was sure that a man had to do the important things by himself.

yourself to be a man. Men are comfortable patting one another on the back, or arm wrestling, or banging into one another on the court or playing field. We are often uncomfortable hugging, or telling our male friends how much they mean to us.

Chowdorow observed that "mothers experience their sons as their male opposite."[26] To define their own identity, boys begin early to separate themselves physically from their mothers. Male development has a clearly defined individuation process. What could be worse for a young male than to have his peers call him a *momma's boy?*

As a male art therapist and teacher I bring to clinical and educational settings a long history of externalization. I bring a deep ingrained belief that my worth is measured by how I perform, how well I have mastered the world. I bring a core belief that vulnerability and intimacy must be approached with great caution. These innate beliefs sometimes cause conflict in my relationships with women students. Sometimes we complement each other. In clinical work, male art therapists will at times be brought closer to their patients because of their masculine traits.

To some degree, the male art therapy student brings each of these aspects of self as well. At times they are problematic, at times they are strengths. There are occasions when the male intern must overcome obstacles that have their foundation in his masculinity. Even so, I believe that the art therapist man is indeed a rare resource to our profession.

To contrast the male developmental experience with that of women, I turn again to my friend and colleague, Deb DeBrular. We co-authored a paper for presentation at the 1989 national conference of the American Art Therapy Association, held in San Francisco. Here are some of her words:

> When I was twenty-three and pregnant for the first time, I hoped and prayed for a boy. Everyone knew I wanted a boy and my parents hoped along with me. They probably had secret concerns that if my baby turned out to be a girl, I would be disappointed. I wanted a boy, not because of any culturally-dictated social order about having a boy first and a girl second; not because of any illusions about creating the perfect family. I wanted a boy because, having grown up as a girl myself, I couldn't see what our culture offered a girl that would make it so nice.
>
> Where I grew up women were seen either as marriage material or sex objects. Being a sex object was bad and offered a future of repeatedly being used by guys who only wanted one thing. Being marriage material was good and offered respect and financial security. If a girl made the decision to be marriage material, she guarded fiercely her reputation. One venture into

erotic behavior could cast her into the role of the sex object, never to return. The journey into eroticism could take various routes. She could lose her head in the back of Joe's dad's car, leaving herself subject to the whims of Joe's advances. Or, the erotic, sexual event could be done against her will. Either way, secrecy was a must.

Wanting the best for their daughter, my parents molded me into marriage material. The script called for secretarial courses in high school, a secretarial job until marriage, then marriage to the right man who would provide for me and our children. Working for a few years before the kids arrived would be tolerated, but no self-respecting man would allow his wife to work, and so after marriage, I would stay at home. My deviations from the script are another story, but at twenty-three and pregnant, life seemed pretty grim.

When I was thirty-five and pregnant again, I wanted a daughter more than anything else in the world. Where years earlier I could define why I had not wanted a daughter, now I wanted one because of some deep, undefinable feeling.

My daughter's arrival was met with joy, but also some sobering thoughtfulness on my part. Here in this precious bundle was a feminine creature who would have me as her role model. I, who hadn't really valued being feminine myself. I had a dilemma. If I could not value being feminine, couldn't value myself, then surely I could not value this tiny female creature. The shock sent me exploring what it meant to be feminine. The exploring led to my profound belief that research being done on the feminine experience is important work that, if not ignored, if we do take notice, will impact every area of our work.

Bruce and I, by virtue of our opposite genders, bring very different things into a relationship, into our therapy groups. What we bring individually has universal qualities. Describing, listing and naming these qualities can possibly be done best by first looking at biology. Our bodies are our first presentations to the world, determining how others will treat us and how we will learn to behave.

What does it mean to be feminine? On the birthing table, the doctor looks to the genitals to determine gender. It is by the hidden nature of the female organs that the doctor and the parents know a little girl has been born. Who can deny the importance of gender when we look at how this first noticed characteristic determines so much of what the child's life will be?

Traditionally, developmental theory has not taken into account the experience of little girls. Male experience has been studied with the assumption that girls do something similar, or as Freud would have it, some strange contorted mirror-image of male developmental theory. More recent work by Nancy Chowderow, Carol Gilligan, Jean Baker Miller, Judith Jordan and others presents the theory that the process of development for girls is very different. Girls are more often raised by primary caretakers of the same sex. The mother and her daughter share the common characteristics of hidden genitals. The daughter comes to know herself as feminine, not through visible evidence, but through the common experience of having something hidden within the body.

A mother experiences her daughter as more like herself. Her relationship with the daughter is characterized by attachment.

Little girls come to relate from this experience of attachment and sharing of hiddenness. Several years ago, I heard a presentation by Jean Baker Miller in which she used the image of an elementary school playground. What are the children doing? The boys are involved in active, competitive games, and the girls are gathered in knots with their best friends, sharing secrets about their relationships.

No little girl in our culture escapes having witnessed thousands of pictures of women scantily dressed, the camera accenting the curves of their figures. It was for this reason that I commented to Bruce early in writing our paper that this was a greater risk for him than for me. Women are accustomed to seeing the female body displayed, but for men to be so exposed is less common. Nudity and exposure are symbols, metaphors, for vulnerability. Part of being a woman is being vulnerable. Not only are we exposed, we are physically smaller. Not only are we portrayed as victims by movies and television, we actually are often victimized in the real world.

When a girl reaches the age of twelve or so, she begins to see physical evidence of her femininity in the reality of her changing body. Biologically, the purpose of the changes that take place in the female body is to provide life to another. The woman's shape becomes the nest, breasts give nourishment. Marie, one of our fourteen-year-old patients, said she believes women must need a softer body because, "they grow babies inside of themselves." The metaphorical theme is one of giving and providing, yet it is a struggle to reconcile the biological purpose with the cultural message.

In her article, *The Human Situation: a Feminine View,* Valerie Saiving discusses the sexual act itself as having for women a passive quality. As she points out, a woman may choose to take an active role in a sexual relationship, but it is not necessary for either reproduction or for bringing satisfaction to her sexual partner. Saiving's interpretation of this phenomenon points to the less competitive nature of women, that assurance of their feminine role is not dependent on performance. Having less anxiety surrounding our sexual role, women are able to place more importance on *being,* in that they have less to prove.

Still, anxiety does exist around the feminine metaphor of sexual intercourse. It is, however, a different metaphor from the male. At Harding Hospital, part of my job was using art processes to assess children and adolescents coming into the acute unit, which opened in 1989. As I observed the issues the young girls brought to the assessment process, one theme recurred. It was concern about intrusion. The girls seemed to be asking, *Will I experience what you do to me as intrusion?*

Many of the girls I saw had been sexually abused, but they are not the only ones who expressed this fear. When I think of the fear of intrusion in light of gender issues and the metaphor of the feminine experience of sexual intercourse, it makes perfect sense.

This is not to say that all sexual intercourse is experienced as an intrusion, but certainly women are always aware of the possibility. While writing this paper, I encouraged Bruce to consider the almost exclusively male act—rape—as one aspect of his presentation. As we talked and processed, it was clearly a struggle for Bruce to think about what to say about rape, about the link between sex, violence and rage. I became frustrated. What I finally realized was that I have thought a lot more about rape than Bruce has. I suspect that women think about rape a lot more than men do.

In considering what I think I saw in my art therapy assessments with young girls—a fear of intrusion—I became aware of how that fear played a part in my negotiating a co-therapy relationship with Bruce. The question has not been the overt, *would Bruce rape me?* but rather the more metaphorical, *would he leave me to be myself? Can I maintain myself in his company?* I suspect I made Bruce feel uncomfortable and on-the-spot more than once over this issue. Not that I ever concretely expressed this fear of intrusion. I leaked enough metaphors, however, that at one point in our pre-group processing, Bruce said to me, "Deb, I will not sexually abuse you." Although at the time this seemed, even to me, a strange thing for him to say, I now believe that sexual abuse is a metaphor for the more subtle, subliminal devaluing of women that happens in our culture.

As a woman I bring this concern about intrusion to the therapeutic process. I bring the feminine history of being devalued and undervalued, and the historical feminine experience of adapting to the subordinate role. I bring my less competitive nature and my comfort with simply *being*. I bring my protection and my nurturance. I bring my desire for strong attachments and my need for relationships to have meaning. All of these aspects of myself can be experienced as problems or as strengths. In honoring our differences, Bruce and I strove to allow them to be strengths.[23]

To illustrate the impact of our developmental differences, our efforts to deal with them in our relationship and the effect this has upon expressive arts therapy groups, I will share a few brief clinical vignettes:

As we walked into the small expressive arts therapy room that morning, the atmosphere was charged with hostile energy. The five severely disturbed adolescent boys, 15 to 17 years of age, had just come from a turbulent community meeting on their unit. During the course of that meeting, several of the nurses had been confronting two of our group members for a variety of aggressive, obnoxious and disrespectful behaviors on the unit. Mumbled epithets cut through the air, "Those fucking bitches" . . . "I'd like to stick something up her ass. . . . " and so on.

The drawing exercise Deb and I had decided upon for the session was, "Cover your page in red and brown, then imagine that it is a section of your own brick wall. What, if any, graffiti would be on the wall?" The boys worked fiercely and the air was heavy with red-brown chalk dust. What emerged graphically were powerful images of rage, expressed in hostile, aggressive, sexualized slogans. Among these: "You are a cocksucker" . . . "Fuck you, cunt" . . . "On the rag" . . . "Eat me, bitch" . . . and the like.

As I turned from my own graffiti and looked at the patients' work, I braced myself for wrestling with the anger and rage that was presented. I looked at Deb's drawing. The contrast was striking. I saw her wall, but I also saw a fragile vine growing up the bricks. For a moment, seeing this small, green life, I was furious with the patients in the group. Inside my head I screamed, *How dare you jerks speak and draw in such a filthy way with Deb in the room?* I was tempted to assume a gallant stance and defend this poor frail vine from the vile creatures that surrounded her. My internal dialogue continued, *To hell with how these kids feel. I have to protect Deb! I have to step in and control . . . even conquer them!* An indignant, self-righteous inner voice exclaimed, *Surely I have never treated a woman so crudely, surely I know how to perform properly with women . . . I've never, ever . . .* and a third inner voice said, *If only Deb weren't here. I know exactly how I'd handle this if it was just us guys in the room.*

In a matter of seconds, all my old tapes about externalizing and performing and solo activity had played within me. I took an emotional step backward and said out loud to the group, "Wow, there is a lot of feeling on the walls today . . . Deb, would you start us off by sharing what you've drawn?"

She began by talking about her wall as being something that protects, but also inhibits her. As she got to the green vine she said, " . . . and I think this vine is about my being a woman. Today I'm really aware that I am the only woman in the group. It seems dangerous in here today." The boys quickly attempted to disavow that their drawings had anything to do with Deb. "It's just those bitches on the unit."

But Deb would not let up. She said, "I hear you say that, but still I see all these angry and sexualized images and I know that women have often been victimized by men. What you do affects me deeply."

The rest of the session was spent in disentangling the violence and sexualized aggression that had been cast on the walls. Several times the group looked to me as if to say, *Explain this to her . . . please.* I resisted the temptation to say, "Aw, come on, Deb, this is just the way guys talk. Don't personalize this." It would have given permission to their behavior.

I believe that each of the boys walked out of that group room on that day with a different sense of male/female relationships for having experienced Deb's vulnerability and my refusal to rationalize their behavior. I could not have brought about that result by myself.

On another occasion, Jan, a woman in her forties, was a relatively new member of our art therapy intern training group, but already her presence was having a curious effect. Clearly, Jan had some issues with me. As weeks passed, Deb and I observed Jan's increasing demand for my attention. She did not seek my approval, or appear needy in any way. No, Jan wanted to fight with me. She was always finding new ways to debate with me.

"Why do you want to fight with me?" I would ask. Jan didn't know, but clearly she loved to hate me. At the same time, it was evident that Deb didn't matter to Jan . . . she was a nonentity.

Outside of the group, the interns buzzed about Jan's seductive behavior towards me. Their conversations and concerns were leaked to Deb and me in various ways as the interns struggled with the intensity of their feelings of competitiveness and anger. It was especially difficult for new members who were trying to understand the task of the group and could not figure out the divisive atmosphere.

In group, masculine symbols began to appear more frequently in drawings, usually in dangerous situations. One woman drew herself slaying a great, half-hidden sea dragon. At first we saw these images as the emergence of issues about men. Later, Deb realized they pertained more to the group's discomfort with Jan's attempts to emasculate me. Her own drawings rigidly, self-protectively repeated stereotypical feminine symbols.

When the conflict was at its peak, Deb and I asked the group to draw how they saw us as leaders of the group. Sharing her drawing, Jan said that she disliked my style, I was too confrontive for her taste, too directive and strong.

When it was Deb's turn to share, she began, "I think my presence is essential in this group right now." She went on to explain to the interns that she knew how to have a relationship with me. "I don't want to change him," she said, "in fact, I like him just fine the way he is. Bruce can be at times very much like the thunder storm, like the lightening that cracks and makes us shiver. I am essential because I know how to have what everyone else in the group seems to want. I am that comforting assurance at the end of the long road through the dark, stormy night."

Probably Jan didn't understand Deb's intervention, but in later groups she was able to focus her energies on issues besides fighting me. The more important result may have been the relief of the rest of the group when Deb contained Jan. They understood perfectly. She had modeled how one woman stays intact in a thunderstorm.

With these vignettes as background, I will explain the process of exploring our relationship in the groups we led. At one time we had three groups: one all male, severely disturbed adolescents; one female adolescent group and the clinical art therapy process/training group. The adolescent patients brought a swirl of complex pathology. The students brought their anxieties, excitement and issues of gender and authority. In different ways, each group challenged our relationship. There were attempts to split us, devour us, idealize, devalue and destroy us.

Deb and I often talked of our relationship as the vessel which contained the group's affect and emotion. I thought of a container made of clay, molded and fired, glazed and strengthened by time. Deb imaged the vessel as flexible and pliant, changing shape with the ebb and flow of group currents.

One image that we agreed upon was the image that lay between us as we met in pre- and post-group discussion. Between us lay a basket, filled with bits of fabric, nuts and bolts, crumpled paper, shards of glass. One of us would pick up some scrap that seemed important. We examined it, got the feel of it, sometimes holding it close and sometimes discarding it as meaningless. These symbolic bits and pieces of past experience were the makings of our relationship. They represented feelings ranging from deep mutual respect to irritation; from warm friendship to disappointment; from laughter to scowls; from tears to silences. Some were history, some in the present tense. We attended to them and in so doing, we attended to the groups we led.

One of our earliest experiences with this basket image happened about six months after we'd begun working as a co-therapy team. We had known each other for six or seven years and felt that our relationship work had already been done. We were mistaken. The adolescent boys group was focusing on how guys treat girls. Confronted by Deb, one of the boys turned to me and challenged, "So what makes you 'n' hers thing such hot shit?"

We resisted the patient's attempt to place us in the role of subjects in the group, but after group we agreed to spend our next supervision session talking specifically about our relationship. Our discussion led us back to our early days, traveled past old hurt feelings and anger, covering our basic admiration of each other and our enjoyment of each other as friends. It was not an easy hour. The self-disclosure seemed endless.

During the very next session of the boys group, the same patient who had challenged us raised again the issue of relationships. This time Deb and I were more ready. This time, the concern floating about the room was not how boys treat girls, it was about how they were treating one another. What began as angry confrontation between two relationship-shy, acting-out macho boys evolved into choked-back tears, drawings of hearts, expressions of feelings for each other and even words of love. I have no doubt that this was the first time in either boy's life he had risked such exposure. Deb and I felt honored to witness the moment.

Such work in the group could not have been done without the work we did in our relationship. Although no mention of it was made in the group, our work together provided an environment of safety that was beyond words.

Despite our conscious efforts to acknowledge our developmental differences and honor them, we sometimes failed to attend to each other. Sometimes I couldn't help acting oppressively; some days I felt manipulated by Deb's passivity. We'd pull something out of the basket that cut or battered us, and for a while we'd bleed and cover our bruises. Although we worked hard at our relationship, it was not a perfect co-therapy team. But we did work.

Deb says, "Our looking at gender issues most affected our art therapy intern group. As young men and women trying to define themselves in relation to their world, our students ran into their own biases and barriers. By being sensitive to the topic, by keeping actively aware of the gender issues between ourselves, we did not neglect, gloss over or bury them at the bottom of our basket."[23]

It is often painful to recognize a need to challenge a system that is centuries old. In our own struggle, Deb and I empathized, understood and contained the pain.

The professions of the creative arts therapies may remain predominantly female. It is essential that in the training situation, whether academic, institutional or clinical, the faculty and supervisors be sensitive to the unique gifts brought by both female and male students. Men and women approach the learning task differently. Female students will come bearing an innate awareness of the value of relationships, intimacy and vulnerability. Male students will bring an appreciation for mastery of technique, skillful performance and individual accomplishment. These different, developmentally-grounded approaches have much to offer each other. It is essential for the health and richness of our discipline that educational programs be aware of and appreciate these differences. The creative arts therapies may lead the way toward providing an atmosphere of honor that will show the polarities of masculinity and femininity to be precious gifts. Not to do so would be to help perpetuate a system that breeds conflict, distrust and political injustice.

Chapter XIII

THE ROLE OF PHILOSOPHY

philosophic, adj. pertaining to philosophy;
* calm, wise and thoughtful.*
philosophize, v. to reason like a philosopher.
philosopher, n. one noted for calm judgment and
* practical wisdom.*
philosophy, n. study of the causes and relations
* of things and ideas; the serene wisdom that comes*
* from calm contemplation of life and the universe.*[10]

(New Concise Webster's Dictionary)

By this point it is no doubt clear to my readers, of either this book or the first, that I am much less concerned with instructing students (or sharing with colleagues) creative arts therapy methods or techniques than I am with discussing philosophies of why we do what we do. Specific creative arts techniques and methodologies must be born and evolve within the context of the individual therapists and their particular clinical settings. This is not to say that the session structures that I employ at Harding Hospital in Worthington, Ohio, would not apply to program settings in Boston, or Topeka or San Francisco, although they may not. My intent is to stress the absolute and universal need for a clear and articulate philosophy of treatment within each and every individual therapist, regardless of location. I do not imply that *my philosophy* must be adhered to, but that *a philosophy* must be present in order for coherent, consistent arts therapy to occur.

In a broader sense this same maxim can and should be applied to treatment units and systems as well. My friend and colleague, Dr. Robert Huestis, the Director of the Department of Psychiatry at Harding Hospital and Unit Director of a long-term adolescent unit, states that "anything that all of the treaters on a given unit agree is beneficial to the patient will be beneficial to the patient"

In my years of clinical work I have been a part of both sorts of

97

treatment programs: those that had a unified agreed upon treatment philosophy, and those in which significant segments of the treatment team were at odds with one another. The relative merits of the two are dramatically evidenced in the progress made by their patients.

Philosophy of treatment must not reside only in intellectual constructs about the nature of a given psychiatric illness, but must embrace a whole range of practical everyday occurrences as well. An example of Dr. Huestis's viewpoint might be that if all members of a treating staff agreed it was important for each patient to start the treatment day with a morning walk out of doors at 7:30 a.m., I believe that 1) this would happen in spite of the resistance one might expect from patients, and 2) that it would in fact be a helpful agent in the life of individual patients. I cite this example purposely because it may at first glance appear trivial and mundane. Yet, when all treaters understand the philosophic grounding of such a structure it will inevitably be of benefit. The potential reasonings behind a 7:30 a.m. constitutional hike might be as follows:

An awareness on the part of treaters that mornings are a predictably difficult time for patients, for a variety of reasons, such as,

A. During sleep the depressed person has had less oxygen going to the brain, exacerbating the depression. It is well known that morning is one of the most difficult periods of the day for the depressed individual.

B. Psychiatric patients often enter treatment with their lives in varying degrees of chaos. The predictable structure of a daily morning walk is a potent meta-message about the need for routine in one's life.

C. The external nature of such a structure is an unspoken metaphor that can be internalized, building and strengthening intrapsychic structure.

D. For the schizophrenic patient the establishment of a daily regimen of routine actions forms the foundation of reality orientation.

E. Such a shared communal task establishes an identification with the notion that therapy is a consistent task that must be worked on daily.

F. For the conduct disordered adolescent this sets the stage for a treatment day willed with learning to struggle with expectations and coping with doing things that you don't want to do, because they have to be done.

I could go on at greater length about a philosophy behind a 7:30 a.m. walk, but I believe you can see my reasoning. For arts therapists there are certainly parallels between such an example and art processes. The art therapist must understand the underlying reasons for, for example, insisting that the schizophrenic patient engage in art processes that reinforce reality orientation by involving repetitive motor tasks. Likewise, the therapist must be clear about why it is more beneficial to the impulsive and entitled adolescent to build his own stretcher frame, to stretch his own canvas and gesso it himself, rather than to buy a pre-stretched, pre-gessoed canvas.

Philosophic, i.e., the calm, wise and thoughtful underpinnings of the myriad details of our work provide the therapist with freedom to move therapeutically within well established parameters. This protects the integrity of the therapy and insures the patient that the therapist is not operating out of a *whatever works or fly by the seat of your pants* approach.

In *Existential Art Therapy: the Canvas Mirror,*[3] I argued that the existential approach provides arts therapists with a profound theoretical and philosophical base from which to work. As an existential art therapist I build my role around three tenets: 1) I do with (and be with) my patients, right where they are, just as they are; 2) I am open and attentive to their lives, and in turn open mine to them; 3) perhaps most important, I bring an attitude of respect and honor to their pain. By doing so I engage them in a process of transformation that brings a radical shift from their position of victim to that of hero. The art psychotherapy process is a journey. I go along as a fellow pilgrim. LISTEN:

Lori was admitted to the short-term child and adolescent unit at Harding Hospital through the psychiatric emergency service. She was fourteen, from a small college town in Southern Ohio. On the night before admission she had attempted suicide by overdose of amphetamines and alcohol.

She had a distinctive style about her. She wore jeans with multiple suggestive tears, a bright red headband and painted black Nikes. She introduced herself as a "skater-hood" who was part of a skate gang. Her first reference to me was in the form of a derisive comment to a peer as I was walking through the unit, "So who's the bald dude?"

On her first day in the expressive art psychotherapy group that I co-lead with Dr. Carol Lebeiko, Lori told us in no uncertain terms that she didn't need to be in this fucking place and that she wasn't about to be in no treatment. My first intervention with her went like this:

"Well, Lori, you're in good company. Look around yourself. No one in this group wants to be in a psychiatric hospital. This is not anybody's idea of an ideal vacation resort."

Dr. Lebeiko then stated our standard introduction to the group. "Lori," she said, "this is a group where we use drawings as a way to get in touch with and share feelings."

Lori snapped, "I can't draw and I don't have any feelings."

Carol continued, "You don't have to be a great artist. Whatever you do will be accepted here. But we do ask that whatever is said in here must stay in here. That way it is safe. And we begin and end every session by checking in with how people are feeling."

With that said, we started our ritual beginning. I asked the group to imagine themselves as some kind of landscape. "Knowing the kind of a person you are, the kind of life you've had, what sort of a landscape would you be?"

The five other patients, Dr. Lebeiko and I stood, gathered chalk, moved to one of the large pieces of paper taped to the wall and began to draw. Lori sat, glaring defiantly. "I can't draw and I don't want to do this crap." Without comment Carol got a box of chalk and gently placed it on Lori's lap.

Carol said, "Just trust your hand, Lori. Whatever you make will be okay."

After a few minutes Lori went to a paper and began to draw. The image that emerged was of a vast empty field, a small clump of weeds in the lower right corner, and a stormy night sky.

When everyone had finished, we sat back in our circle of chairs and began to tell the stories of the landscapes on the walls. As one boy spoke of his raging sea I noticed Lori talking and laughing under her breath, to the girl sitting next to her. I interrupted the boy's story. "Brian, how does it make you feel to have Lori and Amy talking while you are sharing your drawing?" He reddened, looked down at the floor and shyly replied, "Oh, it's okay. I don't really mind."

I put my hand to my head and exclaimed, "But, Brian, you should mind. It's not okay, not okay at all."

Lori reacted, "You don't really expect us to take this shit serious, do you?" She laughed.

"Well, Lori, one thing I know about everybody in this group is that you all have a long history of people not taking your feelings seriously. In this group Dr. Lebeiko and I promise always to pay attention."

She groaned, "Give me a break. These are just stupid pictures. They don't mean a thing."

Carol said, "Bruce and I believe that everything we create is a self-portrait. We take it very seriously."

The group was very quiet. Lori looked around for some support for her resistance, but found none. After a few minutes of silence I suggested we return to Brian's sea.

When we got to Lori's desolate and stormy landscape, she said, "I still don't think this means anything!"

I said, "Yowsa, I am fascinated by this place you've drawn. I can almost hear the wind . . . feel it on my face."

Lori sneered, "Be careful you don't get blown away."

I responded, "Oh, Lori, I've been in lots of stormy places. I'm interested in yours, but I'm not afraid of it."

Carol said, "It must be hard on those plants in the corner."

"They're just weeds," Lori said.

Carol replied, "They look like they could be blown away."

Lori, looking at her drawing, said, "Maybe they should be. They're just trash."

Melanie, a girl who had been in the group for a few sessions, asked, "Do you ever feel that way, Lori? I mean that's a little like how you said your dad makes you feel . . . "

That was all it took. Lori's tough bravado crumbled. Tears welled up in her eyes. She looked away. Again the group was magnificently quiet.

"It's okay, Lori, you don't have to say any more. I think everyone in the group has heard you . . . we understand, we believe you," I said.

Lori was in the group for another three weeks, six sessions. During that time the walls were covered with scenes of her loneliness, brought on by her mother, who had abandoned the family several years before. Fires of rage burned as she depicted her father's alcoholism and abuse of her. Lori was by no means cured by her brief hospitalization; but she did, perhaps for the first time in her life, experience the deep relief of being understood and taken seriously by adults. Carol and I attended to and honored the deep pain and self-loathing she felt upon admission. The pain eased and the loathing lightened.

During her hospitalization, Lori mustered the courage to confront her father. She demanded that he seek treatment for his alcoholism. As fate would have it, he complied and at last report their lives were going much better, one day at a time. Lori's suffering found meaning. As she put it, "If I hadn't tried to kill myself, my dad and I couldn't live together."

Lori's last drawing portrayed her weeds transformed into a rose bush. There were plenty of flowers and a healthy dose of sharp thorns as well. Likewise, Lori's concentration camp has become a home.

The basic tenets of existentialism are that pain, frustration, guilt, loss, loneliness and anxiety, all aspects of human anguish, are unavoidable for human beings. Further, existential writers are skeptical of materialism and hedonism. Recurrent themes are that struggle, suffering and anguish are not only inescapable, but that the individual's efforts to cope with them form the basis of an authentic, full and potentially noble existence.

As an art psychotherapist I am well acquainted with the anguish, suffering and struggle of my patients. As an existentialist I am equally familiar with my own inner turmoil. This is the historic dwelling place of the artist and the figurative home of many disturbed people I've treated.

An existential philosophical base, integrated with my background in the arts and professional experience as an arts therapist, gives me a unique, solid perspective in treating my patients. Throughout time, the artists of the world, painters, dancers, playwrights, poets, have abandoned the pursuit of monetary success and material comfort in their quest for values and truths that go toward the depths of human existence. It has always been the artists of a culture who seek the meaning of life.

My philosophical base offers an opportunity to be with my patients in the midst of their anguish, not for the purpose of making it go away, but in an effort to find the meaning of their pain and bring a sense of honor to their circumstance.

The arts therapist who works from a clearly articulated philosophy, whatever its *brand,* has a framework for understanding, coping with and treating patients. Training programs, as well as treatment programs, must make serious, intentional efforts to develop and communicate their philosophy. As Neitzche said, "He who has a *why* to live for can bear almost any *how*" To paraphrase that for this context, I would say, "He who has calmly thought through *why* he does what he does will surely understand *how* to do it wisely."[28]

TEAMWORK: INTEGRATION VERSUS EXCLUSION

In an article titled *Training the Creative Arts Therapist: Identity with Integration* (Dianne Dulicai, Ronald Hays and Paul Nolan, *Arts and Psychotherapy*, Vol. 16, 1989, pp 11–14,)[27] the authors inadvertently delineated a prominent area of concern within the creative arts therapy profession: "... (a) the graduate must be a competent team member and be able to maintain a professional and competent identity as a therapist; ... " Emphasis must be placed on the "team member" phrase. Most art therapy positions nationwide are in a multi-disciplinary team context. It is imperative that educational programs prepare students for this rewarding and challenging professional milieu.

Unfortunately, all too often students are prepared to be in conflict with fellow team disciplines. Dulicai, Hays and Nolan go on in their article to say, "Current mental health clinical practice requires a level of sophistication beyond the technician-oriented activities therapist model." This statement belies an arrogant devaluation of other disciplines which does nothing to genuinely elevate the creative arts therapies professions. As creative arts therapists we must cease our efforts to compete with psychiatrists, social workers, nurses, occupational therapists, horticulture therapists, psychologists, etc. Maneuvers that seek to define ourselves as equal to, or better than another profession are self defeating and petty. The arts are integrating processes that thrive on the value of divergent materials and flourish on the respectful incorporation of different perspectives. I am deeply appreciative of the lessons I have learned from Carol Dorton, an O.T. assistant, and Chris Burkley, a therapeutic recreation supervisor and Kelly Hunter-Rice, a general activity therapist. These people and many more have taught me the value of the sophisticated therapy that happens in the greenhouse, the craft shop and on the basketball court. Their lessons are every bit as valuable as those I've garnered from psychiatrists, psychologists and social workers. After all, the aim of all these disciplines is to help the patients, to ease their pain.

Many of my colleagues object to being referred to as an *adjunct.* I would argue that if there is genuine team treatment being applied to the patient, all members of the team are adjunct to one another. The psychiatrist is adjunct to the social worker, who is adjunct to the art therapist, who is adjunct to the recreation therapist, etc., etc.

In the graduate level educational training programs for the arts therapies professions, we must prepare therapists who are skilled not only in performing their clinical tasks, but who are also skilled in communicating and participating with doctors, nurses, psychologists and social workers. We must emphasize the importance of teamwork, in which one discipline is not in competition with the others, but rather in concert with them. In sports it is essential that all members of a team work together toward their goals. In therapy it is likewise necessary that each member of the team work collaboratively with colleagues toward the end of restoring mental health to the patient.

As educators we can begin to lay the groundwork for authentic cooperation by eliminating our devaluing references to other activity disciplines. We can also help to formulate positive self-regard in our students by avoiding over-valuing references to physicians and psychologists. We must keep in mind the integrative quality of the arts processes. By doing so we can counteract the disciplinary snobbery so often apparent in the profession.

The educator in creative arts therapies programs must provide the student with a sense of professional identity and self-confidence based upon the unique gifts that arts therapists can bring to the clinical setting. This is done through the role modeling of professors, mentors and supervisors. The role model must be careful to give the student an image of positive professionalism that acknowledges and respects the contributions of a wide variety of therapy disciplines. The educator should avoid definitions of the field that criticize or belittle others.

It has been my experience that from time to time with a given patient, the housekeeper, maintenance man or cook may be of great benefit. The creative arts therapist should be a leader in understanding and validating such contributions. To be a competent team member implies having a healthy regard for all other members of the team. Again, as educators and practitioners of the creative arts therapies it is essential that we remain faithful to the integrative metaphor of the arts processes. By doing so we will ally ourselves and our trainees with a positive celebration of inclusiveness.

Chapter XIV

THERAPY AND HOLIDAYS

An area of consideration that is seldom written about in relation to creative arts therapists, and for that matter all psychotherapies, is the effect of holidays on patients and therapists. My thoughts on this subject have sprung from nearly two decades of clinical experience in an inpatient psychiatric setting. However, I believe that the principles that have evolved are applicable to partial hospital programs. They have been useful in my private practice as well.

I will begin this discussion by looking at some of the difficulties that may arise at special times. Most prevalent and counter-therapeutic ways of dealing with patients during the holidays are:

1) **Denial.** A culturally doomed attempt to ignore the occurence of a holiday, typified by the professional who insists on maintaining a "business as usual" approach, in spite of the mass of social, personal and cultural pressures upon.

2) **Overcompensation.** An attempt to produce an ideal holiday within the therapy milieu.[29]

Both of these approaches are based upon false premises, and in a sense, both are forms of denial. Since denial can never be the servant of reality, these approaches often generate un-authentic encounters between therapists and patients. At best, such interactions provide no therapeutic growth. At worst, they promote regressive feelings, alternately Pollyanna-sweet and bitterly hostile.

To counteract potentially harmful and obstructive interactions between therapists and patients, it is imperative to understand the difficulties that holidays can raise for both. Patients and treaters often have a sense that holidays offer an opportunity or rationalization for taking a break from treatment. The pulls for a therapy-vacation are powerful, magnified because they occur in both parties. Responsible, mature therapists must fight the urge to withdraw from difficult work with patients. This is not the time to schedule a vacation. Therapists certainly need time away from their demanding and often painful routines. However, holiday seasons are not good times for extended absences from one's patients. In the best of circumstances the patient experiences the therapist's vacation as traumatic abandonment. The feeling is intensified and multiplied during special times of the year. It is important that creative arts therapists contain their personal longings for holiday vacations in service to their patients. It is of course crucial that they schedule time away from work at other appropriate opportunities.

Having said that, it is equally important that therapists not assume responsibility for the real or perceived emotional pain their patients may experience during special times. Therapists must maintain their professional and personal boundaries and allow patients to feel whatever they feel.

Holidays, particularly the Thanksgiving, Christmas, Hanukkah season, are stressful for everyone. Cultural images of idealized happy families bombard us and create an expectation of harmony that is unreal and can exacerbate tensions. People in therapy are often in strained family circumstances, and this is heightened during this period. Therapists must stay focused on the reality of the *patient's* life and not project their own experience of holidays and family onto the patient.

At the same time, one can expect that patients' transferences to therapists may be intensified during the holidays. Few if any of my patients have had pleasant and positive experiences with these special occasions. Rather, their dysfunctional families became even more dysfunctional. Certainly a telltale statement such as, "It's (Christmas)—the only day of the whole year that my family can get along," sends warnings that the holiday will be difficult.

Therapists must be wary of their own desire to gratify patients, to make them happy, in order to make themselves happy on the holiday. This is a dangerous temptation. Such occasions test the boundaries of patient/therapist relationships. If boundaries become blurred there is always a significant disruption in the therapy process. Boundaries must be maintained in order for the patient to remain safe enough in the relationship while trying to cope with the season.

To find a middle ground between denial and overcompensation, the holiday must be recognized, but in a way that is clearly separate from the patient's earlier experience. Patient units must establish their own system of traditions that match the realities of patient experience of being hospitalized during the holidays. Creative arts therapists often lay the cornerstones for such tradition development because of their particular sensitivity to the role of image and ritual within the therapeutic milieu. The individual art therapist working in private practice must also make efforts to solidify his or her own sense of celebrative traditions in order to maintain the boundaries clearly.

The lesser holidays such as Halloween, Labor Day, Memorial Day present fewer problems in therapy. They are generally short, in that they do not expand into an entire season. Therefore they are less disruptive to the therapy process and require less special planning on the part of therapists. But even these lesser days demand some measure of forethought. It is again important that the holiday not be ignored, but rather explored for its particular meaning and potential for familial or personal historical significance.

For all therapists, working independently or as part of a treatment setting team, the Thanksgiving—Christmas—Hanukkah season provides a much more complicated and tumultuous set of difficulties. There is no doubt that this holiday season is fraught with cultural and familial expectations that often serve to intensify and magnify pain, anxiety and guilt. It is essential that therapists plan well in advance to explore feelings, expectations and fears about this holiday season with patients before the intense feelings arise. The therapist has a good opportunity to make clear his or her policy (or the institutional policy) about the giving and receiving of gifts among patients and therapists or patient families and therapists. It is recommended that therapists avoid the exchange of gifts with patients or families, for such encounters tend to alter the essential relationship. It is easier to say than to do, but it is my experience that very little good can come from such atypical interactions, and that much bad is possible. Art therapists can save themselves and their patients much discomfort and anxiety by making the boundaries of the relationship very clear well in advance of the holiday pressures.

An important factor here is the element of *specialness* in relationship. Therapists must often contend with their own inner wish to see themselves as unique in the lives of their patients. The wish has a powerful, seductive undertow. We arts therapists tend to see ourselves as creative, special individuals anyway. Further, I suspect that most therapists view their work as a significant and special influence in the lives of their patients. It is not surprising that many receive gifts. Beyond that, many in the creative arts professions feel that they are underpaid, giving persons who deserve being given to. I do not wish to imply that this is a conscious belief, but rather an underlying sense. From the patient or patient's family viewpoint there may also be an unspoken wish to concretize a special bond with the therapist, which is confirmed symbolically by the giving of a gift.

I experienced one example of the complex nature of this dynamic with the parents of an adolescent with whom I had worked for over a year in my private practice. The therapy had gone very well and many of the self-defeating and hostile behaviors of my patient had been worked through. I believe the parents genuinely and consciously wanted to express their appreciation of my efforts with their daughter. The gift they brought me was a bottle of wine. Certainly in our culture this is an often-given gift. However, many of the issues that the patient and I had explored through her art were related to her father's drinking. The gift of a bottle of wine, therefore, took on potent symbolic overtones of malevolence. Since the parents chose to give me the wine in the presence of their daughter, it made for a complicated therapy drama.

I could see that my patient was watching intently for my reaction. I chose to handle this awkward, yet poignant moment by thanking the parents and commenting on the quality of their selection. I added, "...but I'm sorry I cannot accept this gift. I really do appreciate your wanting to give me something, but I think it's most important that giving and receiving takes place in the therapy, between your daughter and me." I did accept the card and again commented that it was a lovely card. The patient's father became angry and left my office without saying another word. The mother was embarrassed and apologized for the father's behavior.

For several sessions after this my patient and I talked about the events of that evening. It was significant that this sparked her entry into an Al-anon group which she eventually got her mother to join as well. The bond that was solidified between my patient and her mother resulted, after some time, in the father entering Alcoholics Anonymous.

As this vignette illustrates, the simple act of giving or receiving a Christmas gift, or refusing to do so, often has far reaching meanings. Had I chosen to accept the gift I would have aligned myself symbolically with the dysfunctional roots of my patient's problems. I had no desire to do that. While the particulars of this example are relatively easy to interpret, I suggest that all such extraordinary exchanges between patients and therapists may have similar potential. Again it is essential that arts therapists have the consequences clearly thought out before they happen.

In summary, it is imperative that therapists think deeply about their relationships with patients during special times. All holidays tend to call up past experiences, childhood memories and family dynamics. Arts therapists must keep their professional focus clearly on the patient, and not succumb to either their own internal drives or external forces that would sidetrack or disrupt the difficult work at hand. There may in reality be no such thing as a free gift with no strings attached. As difficult as it sounds, the work of therapy takes no vacations.

Chapter XV

METAVERBAL THERAPY

As the interns in our training program approach the time for their first solo experience as an expressive arts therapy group leader, one recurrent fear is expressed: *What if I run out of things to say?*

I am always caught in a dilemma of feeling as this fear is voiced. On the one hand I am amused, for I am often overwhelmed by the therapeutic material contained in patients' images. There is always so much that could be said, but not enough time to say it in one group session. On the other hand, the fear-question is frustrating because I have put so much effort into establishing the tenet that the most significant things happen between the artist/patient and the image she creates, and that from this perspective, nothing needs to be said at all. I tell the students over and over, *our words are only the icing on the cake.*

The intern's question, humorous and irritating as it is, speaks to a central issue in the creative arts professions. How much of what we do can, or should, be put into words? Arts therapies are often described as *non-verbal* modalities. This defines the field through the negative. I have chosen to work in a *metaverbal* framework, from a viewpoint that the arts therapies go *beyond words.*

When asked to explain the distinction, I ask my students to remember a significant event in their lives. Some recall a birthday, others a wedding, others the death of a family member. In each case I ask them to describe what happened. Students share memories of people, things they did, the place they were, and so on. Then I ask them to recount specific conversations from these significant events. Invariably it is difficult, if not impossible to do. Where descriptions of people and actions were rich, full of life and color, the verbal recitations are sparse and difficult to reconstruct. My point in this exercise is that most people retain images longer than they retain words. I am also convinced that life's deeper moments and more meaningful experiences are nearly impossible to put into words.

An example for me was the births of my children. After the events, I tried to tell anyone and everyone who would listen all about these miraculous happenings and my feelings about them. As hard as I tried to convey the depth, the awe, the mystery, I still felt that my words were inadequate. Now, looking back, I cannot recall anything being said in the birthing room at all, but I have vibrant images of holding my son and daughter for the first time.

In our culture we are bombarded by words. We see them on signs, in the newspaper, books and magazines. We hear them on the radio, television, and in conversation. There are so many words in just one day. It is impossible to retain. The sheer volume of words have rendered them impotent.

We can only imagine what it must have been like when the primitive man or woman first uttered a sound meaning *water* and was understood by another. What power, to speak the name of water and call up the image of water in the mind of another! The word was the symbol, the embodiment of the thing it represented. *Word* is derived from the Greek *logos*, which referred to the controlling principle of the universe as manifested in speech. In Christian theology, *The Word* is the eternal thought of God made incarnate in Jesus Christ.

When examined from these perspectives, words have rather a different weight than is currently given them. It may well have to do with their early connection with *image*. The image-words of fire, water, beast or food had much to do with the ultimate concerns of primitive man, i.e., survival. Today words are often used to disguise, euphemize and obscure real meaning.

I am convinced that the real substance of our work as creative arts therapists takes place between the patient, the media and the process. What we say about this interaction in no way alters the nature of the process. Our words may serve to validate (for the therapist) the meaning of the process, but they do nothing to change the meaning itself. In a radical sense, I believe it would be possible for arts therapists to do our most significant work without speaking at all.

In the hospital or clinic setting, there are many professional disciplines whose primary way of relating to the patient is through verbal interaction. Our special gift to the treatment of patients is that the arts provide a meta-verbal arena in which to form a relationship.

I encourage my students to regard with skepticism their desire to talk with the patient. The wish to say the *right thing* or the fear of saying the *wrong thing* may represent a distrust of the artistic process.

When the student worries, *what if I run out of things to say,* one can only respond by encouraging the student to trust the image. This may be difficult, since educational systems rely so heavily on words. If the educator attempts to teach an approach that does not depend upon the skillful manipulation of words, he or she must wrestle with finding new methods of instruction.

I have already challenged the need that many art therapists have to talk with patients about their images. I firmly believe that we could do most of our work with patients without speaking at all. However, it is a reality that the mental health professions depend heavily on words to describe the therapeutic work in process. Certainly most practicing art therapists and students must function in institutions or in treatment settings that are predominantly populated with colleagues from verbal disciplines. Still, I want us to work and think together about images and about language. For those students who will soon be out in the world treating patients, this is an important subject. All of your good work with patients may come to nothing if you cannot put into words what you and your patients experience together. Insurance companies may not pay for your work and your employers may not take you seriously if you cannot articulate what you do.

This is tricky business, for I believe that the best of what happens between me and my patients and their artistic images is beyond description. It's a lot like trying to find words to describe making love with my wife, or being hugged by my children or watching them compete in a game. There are few words to describe such happenings in our lives.

Poems, dramas, dances, sculptures, paintings and drawings are not mere intellectual constructs. They are glimpses of the inner life of human beings, snapshots of internal reality. Each pencil line, every dissonance and every spot of color are announcements to the self and to the rest of humanity that *I am.* The artist, in whatever medium, proclaims to the world, *I have something to say.*

The overall *gestalt* of an artwork is often indescribable in words. Just what did Hopper mean to say in *Nighthawks?* What exactly was E.E. Cummings trying to tell us in *Anyone Lived in a Pretty How Town?* Such questions inspire lengthy argument, but I am wary of any who claim to know the answer. The configuration of the artist as a biological, social, cultural, familial, internally and externally dynamic creator is overwhelmingly complex. Perhaps the most that the audience or the beholder can do is to catch a wisp of the multifaceted communication of the creator. From such glimpses come the first fumbling words of a dialogue between the artist and the beholder. As we arts therapists view the works of our patients, we must struggle to find words that focus the expressed thought, the feelings, the physical effort and the soul of the artistic product. Always approach a piece of art with a sense of reverence for the story that has been told, as mysterious as it may be. Each time a patient scrawls images across the page with chalk, each time she struggles with pen in hand to find the next line of her poem, each time the child dabs a brush and smears it across the paper, it is proclaimed to the world, *I know something, I have something to say.* Inwardly, they wonder, *Will anyone listen, will anyone understand?* As we approach the proclamations, we must respect their sacredness and earnestly seek dialogue with the images.

Originally words were powerful enough to instigate action or call up images essential for survival. One needs only witness the first word of a child: *Mama.* The child speaks the name of that which is essential for its own safety and flourishing. What a powerful word this is. Words have also come to be a means of creating distance from one another and removing ourselves from the experience of life. In its origins, the practice of psychotherapy was described as the "talking cure." However, psychology has become ever more concerned with the use of words that limit, define and constrict experience rather than those that broaden expression.

The Missouri saying, "show me" embodies our skepticism of words. We long for observable facts, measurable data and quantifiable results. We have, nearly, lost the ability to reason imaginatively. Our language and thinking, heavily influenced by the scientific method, have become linear and fact-oriented. In the psychotherapeutic professions there is a tendency to find words that will describe, contain and make understandable. As we try to describe our patients' illnesses and explain their pathological behaviors, we often leave no room for the imaginal, the ambiguous and paradoxical. Metaphorical glimpses and wisps of insights have become antithetical to the scientific method. It is as if we believe that if we can explain, if we are knowledgeable enough and if our language can somehow accurately describe, then we will be in control.

In my first book I described the phenomenon of imagicide; that tendency we all have to want to confine, define and constrict the images of another. To do so is to kill the power of the image. Whenever I try to explain another's image, I delude myself that by describing their image, I will somehow be knowing them in a deeper way. In fact, my explanations take me further from their experience. The more I try to grasp the meaning of Beth's image intellectually, the further I remove myself from it. I must sit and be still and be with her.

All of us in the western world have been taught to seek that which can be proved through reason and scientific method. We have been instructed to be wary of spirits and souls and ambiguous forces. Therefore we tend to compartmentalize things, to put things into categories: right and wrong, good and bad, thoughts and feelings. Our culture has a hard time appreciating the paradox of something that is *both* good and bad, or even *between* good and bad.

As an art therapist I believe that the images of my patients, no matter how painful, horrific or frightening, are expressions not of pathology and sickness, but rather of movement toward help. The art making does not create the image within the patient; it frees it. It brings the dark, painful and monstrous into the light. It is survival, a celebration of life. Patients reach deep within themselves and bring out their pain, their illness, their courage. The art therapist does not see what is wrong, but sees the images that are transforming the self. They need to be there, the art therapist needs to be with them. We hardly need to talk at all.

The language I use in the presence of my patients and their images is not definitive. It is the language of metaphor. My words serve to attach me to the patient and the image. My conversation only validates publicly that I am here, I have seen and I will stay.

Over the past 17 years I have developed some measure of proficiency in using the clinical language of the psychiatric milieu. I can speak with confidence of diagnostic categories from DSM III R. I can converse about symptoms and observable behaviors. I know how to write clinical charts that will be acceptable to third party payers, and I can talk with my psychiatrist friends about a variety of psychiatric theories and treatment approaches. Clinical language is the meeting-ground for the helping professions, but it is incomplete. I prefer the lively language of the image. Sometimes I stumble among my words. Other times, my peers look at me as if I am speaking a foreign tongue. It is not easy to speak as an art therapist. There is no well-defined comfortable professional facade. But it is preferable to the imagicidal alternatives.

The original purpose of words was to evoke images. In the clinical setting I am an archeologist of language. I carefully dig through the verbal debris, searching for the long lost image. I look to poetry, fables and metaphor. I look for words that are alive with an expressive power of their own. I learn from the language of religions long gone and from dreams, and from the rock-and-roll lyricists of today. I struggle to find words that will allow the image to speak through me. I make no attempt to speak for the image.

It is essential for all art therapists, whether seasoned practitioner or novice, to hold in tension the polarities of language. No words will ever adequately describe or contain a work of art. In order to function in the treatment world, we must find words that will enable others to glimpse the metaverbal nature of our work.

Chapter XVI

THE MIRROR

In *Existential Art Therapy* I used the image of "the canvas mirror"[3] as a metaphor of the introspective process that I believe is the foundation of art making. "There have been periods of my life when I have looked into the mirror and found images of courage and integrity. I have also seen open wounds, loneliness and cowardice . . . When I try to run from the canvases' reflection I am intensely aware that I am running . . . there is no escape" (Fig. 16).

The image of the mirror has emerged again for me. It is not intended as clever literary consistency from book to book, but rather as a clear affirmation that self-reflection and transparency are cornerstones of our work as creative arts psychotherapists and as creative arts therapy educators.

As I prepare to lecture at various training programs around the country, I always ask the faculty to describe the nature of their relationship with the students. I want to know if my approach to education will be consonant with what the students have already experienced. My colleague, Shaun McNiff, summarized *Existential Art Therapy* by saying he felt as if he'd been invited into a confessional cell. The thought had never occurred to me that what I wrote would be read as being that intimate. Reflecting on his feedback, it became clear to me that this describes in some ways my position as an educator. I have no interest in teaching from a detached stance of intellectual objectivity. I do not believe that therapy of any sort can be taught or learned that way.

There must be elements of intellectual objectivity, of course, but that is not enough. The student must be both *studied* and *studier*, the object and subject of inquiry. The same is true for the educator. The teacher must be both the form and the content of presentation. The mentor must do more than cite appropriate references, must be willing to be the focus of critical research and interrogation from the student. This is not easy work—*it ain't for sissies.*

My colleague, George Gibbs, who is the Chaplain at Harding Hospital, criticizes the tendency of authors of "therapy books" to present only their

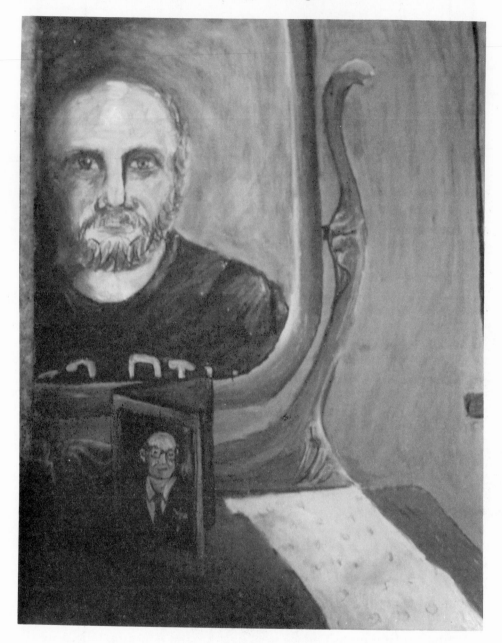

Figure 16. I have seen images of courage and cowardice.

success stories. As promoters of a point of view or philosophy, we authors seldom mention the patient we failed to help, the patient who resisted our best efforts at benevolent assistance. I think George's point is well taken, and would include myself as one of the "success storytellers." I will do it again in this book, for I am arguing for a point of view. If pushed for a label for this perspective, I would say I am an arts therapy educator. What is more, I am an arts-therapy-as-sacred-task educator. Still, I would not want to imply that my approach is always successful. I have tasted the bitterness of failure.

Chapter XVII

FAILURE

O ver the past seventeen years, I've been involved directly in the hospital treatment of twelve or so human beings who despite my best efforts and the efforts of many others, are now dead. They died by their own hands. These remembered names and faces are dramatic testament that there are failures in this work. Sometimes the psychotherapy, art psychotherapy, psychopharmacology, intensive nursing care, sophisticated psychological testing, adjunctive therapies and family therapy all added together equal zero, that is, no therapeutic change whatsoever.

While the suicide of a patient with whom you've worked closely is graphic evidence of failure, there are many more subtle failures that we treaters must endure. We are not gods.

Ultimately it is the patient who does the hardest work in therapy. It really is their success when the therapy works and their failure when it does not. Still, we would-be healers cannot divorce ourselves from our own pride in effective work and disappointment in unsatisfactory progress.

Probably 95% or more of the case study literature in our field deals with therapeutic success. This is understandable. No one relishes having students or peers read about their failures. Yet this is unfortunate, for the reality is that many people who seek psychotherapy, regardless of form, do not improve as a result of their therapy. Some people get worse, some make no change at all. Fortunately, many get better.

The focus of this chapter is failure. It is not an easy chapter to include, but it is an essential aspect of the arts therapy professions. It is important that students know that there will be times in their professional lives when they will feel badly about their work. They will be frustrated by their own impotence. They will be wounded from time to time by their inability to make someone change. We practitioners must be more open about this. There is little hope for our own healing if we do not own our scars.

I include here a vignette of failure. It represents a composite picture of a host of failures. They are my failures, my colleagues' failures and my patients' failures. There have been many, and no doubt there are many more to come.

What To Do About Jane

Jane was twenty-four when I first met her. She'd been referred to my private practice by a psychiatrist from a large general hospital. She was quite depressed and had been unresponsive to the psychiatrist's verbal and medical interventions. She had recently been in a car accident. Her father had died about six months before her first visit to my office.

During her first session she completed a large chalk drawing which she titled, *My Inner and Outer Worlds.* She covered the page in black, then smeared blue across the black background. The emotional tone of the drawing was depressing and bleak. In a variety of ways I tried to explore with Jane the meaning of this black and blue portrait of self. I worked very hard in that first session. In retrospect, Jane worked hardly at all. It was as if she presented this dark image and then disowned it.

At the close of the session I encouraged her to keep her drawing, to take it with her.

Bruce: Maybe you should save this. It may be the first part of our journey together.

Jane: I don't want it. You'd better keep it for us.

Bruce: Are you sure? I know it represents hard feelings, but someday you may wish you'd kept it.

Jane: No, I don't have any place in my apartment to store it. You can keep it, or throw it away.

In this small interchange, Jane had subtly set the parameters of our relationship. In a sense, she had written the contract that I was to fulfill. It would be my job to take care of, to hold, to store and dispose of her bad feelings. She did not have room for them.

Unfortunately, I did not pick up this message clearly until nearly eighteen months had passed. During that time, Jane created a host of images related to her negative self view, the tragedies of her life and the mistreatment she received at the hands of others. She would draw or paint these and then dump them on my floor, soliciting my prescription.

An example: She drew herself and her roommate engaged in a heated argument about getting up in the morning. Jane had somehow got her roommate "responsible" for awakening her in time for work. She told the story that her roommate was always harsh in the morning and that she (Jane) resented being awakened so rudely. The picture was filled with two angry mouths casting fire towards each other.

I suggested that she might buy an alarm clock and get herself up. Jane obediently did so, but came in the following week furious that her roommate had not been reminding her in the evening to set her alarm clock. She had been late for work on two occasions. Her boss was angry with her and she was angry at her roommate and at me.

In the course of her therapy Jane presented situation after situation like this. I began to set aside time in my schedule before her appointments so that I could prepare for Jane's visits. I began to dread her appointments.

After some time it occurred to me that I was working a whole lot harder on Jane's therapy than she was. Once this became clear to me, I was able to develop what I considered to be a more coherent strategy for dealing with her. My plan was to do less.

As Jane entered my office she said, "It's been a horrible week. I've felt so bad I haven't been able to go to work. I haven't worked on my journal, haven't painted. I haven't been able to do anything."

Bruce: Sounds bad.

Jane: So what do you want me to do today?

Bruce: I don't know, Jane.

Jane: What do you mean, you don't know?

Bruce: I don't know what you should do, Jane.

Silence

Jane: (angrily) What is this? You're supposed to help me, not just sit there. You're acting like my old counselor.

Bruce: How am I like him?

Jane: You're not doing anything to help me.

Bruce: What do you want me to do, Jane?

Jane: I don't know. Tell me to draw something or ask about my journal. Something!

Bruce: Well, Jane, I am doing, and have been doing something for a long time now. I've been here with you, I've never missed an appointment. For that matter, you've really accomplished a lot, too.

Jane: Like what?

Bruce: Well, you've maintained our relationship for a year and a half. It hasn't been easy, but you've stuck with it.

Jane: But I still feel like crap.

The rest of the session continued in much this same way. Jane called and canceled the next session. She rescheduled but failed to keep the next appointment. About six weeks went by before she called again. She wanted to tell me that she'd decided that she needed a new therapist and that she'd found a "wonderful woman psychiatrist" whose office was in her neighborhood.

I suggested that we might meet at least once more in order to bring our work together to a close. Jane coolly declined, saying that she saw no reason for such a meeting.

I have since met her psychiatrist and learned that Jane went to only a couple of sessions with her and then decided that she needed other help than the psychiatrist was willing to provide. So it goes.

This was a disturbing failure for me as a therapist. Not only was I unable to help Jane make the changes she needed, but the relationship I had so thoughtfully nurtured ended in such an abrupt and unclean manner that it raised questions about the relationship all along. Did we ever really have a relationship? How could she terminate the therapy in such a way? Was I completely fooled? What could I have done differently? How . . . what . . . why . . . should? These questions plague me as they plague all would-be healers. Was it my failure, or Jane's failure, or our failure, or no one's? Or, was this experience just a blip in Jane's long history of necessary treatment in her life? I do not know, and for now I must be content with my inability to know.

As an educator in the field, I see it as my responsibility to guide my interns toward a realistic sense of the profession. I believe that it is essential to help them develop a real view of the work. A real view includes the fact of failure.

In the medical world doctors must contend with their own finite capabilities. The ultimate reminder of this is the death of their patient. It is one of the tragedies of medicine that technology has fostered an unreal denial system for the physician. Even with the most sophisticated life support systems available, eventually, ultimately, inevitably the patient dies.

We arts therapists have no such technology. Likewise, we do not generally hold life in our hands. Still the analogy is apt. Ultimately the work of getting better is the patient's work to do. Many will and many will not. This represents a paradoxical situation for the therapist. What we do is incredibly important, but all we could do is not enough.

My friend, Dr. Henry Leuchter, used to tell me, "Bruce out of every ten people you meet, two are going to like you no matter what you do. Two are not going to like you no matter what you do. The rest are up for grabs." Perhaps this is the way it is with patients as well. Two will get better no matter what you do. Two will get worse. . . . The rest are up for grabs.

Chapter XVIII

THE ROLE OF METAPHOR

Not long ago a young man was referred to an expressive art psychotherapy group. In requesting the consultation, the physician explained that the patient had been in individual psychotherapy for three
months and in the long-term treatment unit for adolescents for more
than four months, but had made little progress because of his very rigid
defenses. Discussing the situation further with the psychiatrist, I learned
that the patient usually avoided his psychotherapy sessions. When he
did attend, he often walked out after ten minutes or so. The psychiatrist
was frustrated by this sixteen-year-old's defiant attitude, which was best
summed up in the patient's words, "Fuck therapy. I want to go home."

The therapist had employed many approaches in an attempt to engage
James. At first he assumed a non-directive manner. When this made no
headway, he became more actively supportive and friendly. This provided James with many opportunities to reject the therapist and devalue
the process. The therapist shifted to a more directive and confrontive
mode, but this too had served only to increase the patient's resistance to
self-exploration and sharing. In short, the patient was stuck in a resistive
stance. His insurance resources were being drained and the treatment
team were afraid that time was running out for James.

James's history included truancy, vandalism, drug and alcohol abuse,
violent behavior with peers and family members. The psychiatrist feared
that James would end up in jail, or dead, if he did not make some
changes in his life. Hospitalization was a "last chance" effort to turn
things around.

As my co-therapist and I discussed James's entry into our group, we
made careful note of the failed therapeutic interventions. We decided
that we would (1) avoid confrontation whenever possible and (2) try
to engage James through the metaphors of his images, whatever they
may be.

In the first session that James attended, we began by instructing the
group members to cover their large (3′ × 3′) papers with red and brown

chalk. They were then asked to smear the colors together, making a solid red-brown surface. James was skeptical and made several quiet, devaluing comments to his peers. However, since everyone else in the group was working at the task, James complied. My co-therapist and I noted his comments but did not intervene or respond to his negativity.

Then I said, "Now what we have here is a segment of a brick wall. Your task is to apply whatever graffiti or slogans or drawings you'd want to put on your brick wall." James seemed to like this idea. It was in some ways vandalizing, which he knew how to do. He quickly picked up a white chalk and wrote, "Fuck therapy." He then drew the anarchy symbol, a smoldering marijuana cigarette, a bottle of beer and a red smear. He told the boy next to him that the smear was a bloodstain from where someone had hit the wall with a fist.

As the group members shared their images, my cotherapist and I, as always, made every attempt to honor the drawings and their content. When James shared his drawing I commented (staying with the metaphor) that it appeared that James's wall had had some very rough experiences.

James: Wha' ya mean?

Bruce: Well, it looks like someone has hit this wall, and I see that the wall has been around drugs and alcohol.

James: Like I always say, fuck this.

(James quickly looked to his peers for support of his challenging attitude.)

Bruce: Well, James, you know in this group we always take things that are drawn very seriously.

James: Don't go bein' therapeutic with me. I just drew this shit. It don't mean anything.

Bruce: It's okay if that's what you think. But I have this idea that what we draw is kind of a portrait of who we are.

(James stared.)

Bruce: Of course, I don't know what to make of this Fuck Therapy stuff. You do realize that this is a biological impossibility?

James: What in hell are you talking about?

Bruce: You do realize that it is not possible to have sexual intercourse with therapy.

At this, James and the other boys in the group began to laugh. My cotherapist and I laughed, too. Then I shifted back to the image.

Bruce: But really, James, I see the blood on your wall and I know
somebody hit you, I mean your wall, pretty hard.

James: Yeah, lots of times. So what?

Bruce: It looks like this is a strong wall, James. I'm glad you have it. It
seems like you have needed your wall to protect you.

James: Yeah, I guess.

This was the beginning of James's journey into himself. Over the next
few months he led us over a path past scenes of abuse from an alcoholic
father, metaphorically depicted as a monster who "steps on baby chicks."
Episodes of destructive sexual acting out were represented in the symbolic forms of animals forced to share a cavern/prison.

As James grew more comfortable in the group and his story became
more apparent through his images, he gradually dropped his hostile,
resistant behavior. He began to take his drawings to his individual
therapist, where he told his tale again. As his old distancing maneuvers
were abandoned he allowed himself to become attached to the nursing
staff, activity therapists and others on the treatment team.

The classic definition of a metaphor is a figure of speech containing
an implied comparison, in which a word or a phrase ordinarily and
primarily used for one thing is applied to another. For our work as
creative arts therapists and educators, this definition is insufficient, for it
ties one to verbal constructs. James's metaphors were not built of symbolic language. They were forged of images made of chalk and paper.
Without them, I do not believe he would ever have been able to benefit
from his hospital stay or make use of therapy.

In *Depth Psychology of Art*, Shaun McNiff suggests "The re-imagining
of the artist is taking place through the work that we are doing today in
the arts and psychotherapy."[14] His first steps in this process took the form
of revisiting the nomenclature of our profession. As necessary and admirable as his effort is, it is curious that he offers only one sentence
regarding metaphor. "Metaphors are images which are used symbolically
for the purpose of comparison, articulation, elucidation." I agree with
him, but I wish he had at least devoted an entire page to broadening this
sentence, or perhaps used **bold type** or <u>underlining.</u> Metaphors are
images. This is the key element, the most potent element of our discipline.

Images are metaphors containing an inherent comparison in which
one thing is used to describe another. James's metaphors, without which

no therapy would have occurred, were his images of monsters and chicks, prisons and caves, walls and graffiti.

As arts therapists, educators and students, we must develop a reverence for the image/metaphor. We must not attempt to imprison it through vocabulary. We must foster a sense of awe and commit ourselves to the notion that the image can, and should *just be.* I do not propose an anti-verbal doctrine; rather I call for a strong pro-meta-verbal faith in image metaphors. If paint is in the veins of this artist-therapist, metaphor is in my heart.

All things we create are partial self-portraits. Any image that comes through us is both itself and a description of its creator. The arts therapist needs only to look and be with the images of the patient. We hardly need to talk at all. As McNiff suggests, the purpose of the metaphor is to elucidate, or make clear.

The need to talk, or put into words, is a phenomenon that often makes me uneasy with colleagues in arts therapy and other disciplines as well. It seems to indicate that the therapist does not trust the image. It is essential that we creative arts therapists *value the clarity of communication that is presented in the object or process* of art making. *We hardly need to talk at all.*

Chapter XIX

THE ROLE OF LOVE

Don't talk of love, I've heard the word
before . . . "[30]

Paul Simon

For the most part, this book is about the training of would-be art therapists in the discipline of the profession. This chapter will explore what lies behind, or perhaps beneath the discipline. We must ask ourselves what is the *motivation,* the *push,* the *energy* for our work. I believe that energy is *love.* I feel a little uneasy saying so. I have looked at many degree-program catalogues, public relations materials from universities and have failed to find any direct mention, or even veiled reference to love. Still, I believe it is the force that pushes us educators, pulls us therapists and seduces students of the profession. Of course I am aware that by attempting to explore love, I will be discussing the immeasurable, illogical and mysterious. As Scott Peck describes, " . . . we will be attempting to examine the unexamineable and to know the unknowable."[28] Even so, I think it is essential that an attempt be made to grapple with this force, for it is surely the foundation upon which most, if not all therapeutic endeavors are built. Therapists receive money for what they do, but it is clear that most of us are not in the game to get rich. There are other more direct routes to that end, ones with fewer headaches and heartaches at that.

Countless works of art, paintings, poems, songs, dances and dramas have as their sole purpose the attempt to define love. They seem, however, only to describe various facets of love. The subject may be too big to be understood and too deep to be confined by language. Greek philosophers reduced the prismatic nature of love to three categories: *agape, philia* and *eros.* In *The Road Less Traveled,* Peck offers a simpler definition: "The will to extend one's self for the purpose of nurturing one's own or another's spiritual growth."[31] This complicates the matter by requiring further definition of *spiritual* and *growth.*

I offer yet another definition of love, with proper acknowledgement that it, too, is an inadequate and clumsy attempt. I define love as *The will to attend, to be with, one's self and the self of others.*

As a creative arts therapist with much personal history with other action-oriented therapies such as occupational therapy, recreation therapy, horticulture therapy and work therapy, I am deeply committed to the maxim, "Actions speak louder than words." Therefore I begin my definition of love with "the will to . . . " By using the word "will," there is an implicit integration of intent or wish and action. Will is a wish so powerful that it must become an act. One cannot simply want to be loving, it must be manifest in action towards others and the self. Will also connotes free choice. To attend to another is an act of choice. I do not have to do it, and in fact there are probably many times that I choose, for one reason or another, not to attend. Paradoxically there are moments, particularly in the art psychotherapy studio, when I am deeply attuned to a patient without my conscious effort. At some deep level I have chosen to openly be with the patient. Thereby I have chosen to love.

Implicit in my definition of love is a quality of give-and-take, a dialogue. It is impossible to be genuinely attentive to another if you are not attentive to yourself. In the context of the art psychotherapy studio, "being with" the images created by the patient enhances one's ability to be with one's own images. This creates an artistic, circular process of loving awareness.

A final comment about my definition of love as the will to attend to one's self and the self of another: although it is an act of will, a choice, the force itself is without a goal or purpose. One loves for the sake of loving; one attends to self or other for the sake of attending. Loving does not bring material gain, or power or prestige. It brings only itself, and that is the mystery.

The patients who come to the creative arts therapist for psychotherapy have often been victimized by those who should have been their most loving supports. They come bearing emotional scars, the remnants of physical, sexual or emotional abuse. They come hungry for attention and yet frightened, guarded and defended from its curative effects. This is why educational programs designed to teach the creative arts therapies must begin to wrestle with love. It is not enough to teach mastery of media, developmental theory, psychotherapeutic technique, third-party payor documentation procedures and the history of the profession. We must begin a dialogue with students as early as possible about the deepest and most noble motivation of the discipline, love.

The creation of art is itself an act of love. As the artist dips the brush into the pigment and moves color to the empty canvas, an image begins its incredible pilgrimage from deep within to without. Lines, shapes and colors are added, the image takes form and is born. There is a continuous push and pull between the artist, the medium and the canvas. The image emerges from imagination, conflict and emotion. The process, this attending to, is deeply moving, so filled with subtle nuance that it cannot be accurately described. The artist alone experiences the full meaning of the unfolding event. It is the task of the art psychotherapist to be with the patient/artist, acting as midwife to the birth of self. The art psychotherapist must love in such moments. Doing so provides a healing, restorative milieu for the patient.

The therapeutic context is a community of love. It may be a community of two—therapist and patient—or a larger community in the case of expressive psychotherapy groups. Existential meanings can be found only through transcending the self. Creative acts can best be appreciated and stimulated in the realm of relationship.

The artist establishes the parameters of her love through the performance of her creative endeavors. She acts out of love as she creates; love of herself and love for the community. The art therapist, through acceptance, praise or confrontation, acts out his love by seriously engaging with the art and its creator.

The mystery of this creative interaction among artist, image and therapist is that such love is neither earned nor imposed. Creation and attention are acts of grace, not forced or deserved. The mystery is felt as one steps away from the canvas in order to get a different perspective. It is sensed in the fleeting moments as the artist signs the work, knowing that the signature does not denote "I did this," but, "I am this." The mystery is present as others pause to look, to see and be with the image.

Being attended to sharpens one's ability to value self and others. Both the loved and the lover see the world with new eyes. All images and actions are enhanced and given meaning through the grace of love. From meaning comes the motivation to create again. From creation comes meaning, comes motivation, comes creation ... on and on the loving goes.

A Digression

Diana had been in the expressive arts psychotherapy group only twice before. The group consisted of seven adolescents from the dual diagnosis unit at Harding Hospital, and myself. Patients admitted to that unit suffered from psychiatric disorders severe enough to warrant inpatient hospitalization and significant drug or alcohol abuse symptoms. This was often a difficult group, resistive and devaluing toward treatment. Complicating matters further, Diana and two of her peers had been ordered into the hospital by the juvenile court system. The general emotional tone of the group was hostile.

On this particular day I'd chosen to introduce the drawing exercise, "the emotional mirror" as the focus of the session. One boy, Dave, who was perhaps the most negative and hostile of the group, drew a large "F." "U." Beside the letters he added a stick figure with a brown pile of horse manure where the head should be. The stick figure held a piece of chalk in one hand. I quickly grasped the overt message to me: "Fuck you, shithead."

Diana and her peers in the group also got the point of his drawing and were snickering and whispering among themselves, no doubt wondering what my reaction would be. Internally, I felt a flash of anger. A voice within me shouted, *How dare you do that in here?* Another interior voice prodded me to confront Dave with the harshest blast I could muster. But a third voice whispered, *What you do in the next few minutes will have real impact on the life of this group. Respond as lovingly as you can, Bruce. Don't react!*

I finished my drawing and sat down, silently surveying the works around me. From each of the seven emotional mirrors fierce and painful images glared back at me. Diana's drawing was a representation of a backseat car window with the bottoms of two feet hanging out. The scene was surrounded by harsh black and purple slashing lines. There seemed to be a red trickle of blood seeping through the crack and the frame of the car.

Since so much attention was being focused on Dave's drawing, I decided to begin the group dialogue with his image.

Bruce: Well, Dave, your drawing seems to have stirred the interest of the group.

Dave: Yeah, so what!

Bruce: Well, it's quite a strong image. Dave, would you like to say anything about it?

Dave: Don't play yer damn games with me, man. I ain't in the mood.

Bruce: I'm not playing games, Dave. I mean it, that is a very strong image. The whole point of being in this group is to express yourself. You certainly did.

Clearly this was not the reaction Dave, or anyone else in the group, had expected to get from me.

Dave: So wha' you gonna do about it?

Bruce: I'm not going to do anything, Dave. I'm just being with it.

Dave: Huh?

Bruce: Dave, you know I believe that everything we create is sort of a self portrait. When I look at your "Fuck You, Shithead" I really get a sense of how you feel about things. It must be really hard.

Dave: What?

Bruce: Really, thanks for sharing with the group. It's a gift, to let people know how you feel about yourself and the world.

Then, without hesitation, giving Dave no time to respond, I asked who would like to share their drawing next. Diana said, quietly, "I'll go." She stared at her image for a few moments.

Diana: I don't know why I drew this. At first, when I saw what Dave was doing, I thought this would be funny . . .

(long pause)

Bruce: And now . . .

Diana: Now I don't know.

Bruce: It doesn't look very funny to me, Diana.

One of the other girls laughed nervously and said, "Looks like Friday night at the Drive-in to me."

Bruce: It doesn't look like very much fun, though. Look at all those lines around the outside. They look violent. And that looks like blood coming out of the door. No, it doesn't look funny, Diana.

I looked from the drawing to Diana. Tears were running down her face, making wet spatters on her blouse. The room was quiet and still.

Diana: I was raped when I was thirteen. (sobbing) Since then I've put my feet up for just about any guy who asked.

From across the room, Dave said, "That really sucks...you're too good for that, Diana. Nobody should treat you that way!

Diana: It's not them anymore. Didn't you hear what Bruce said about your drawing, Dave? It's me! It's how I treat me. (more sobbing)

One of the other group members fidgeted in her seat, "Can we go on now?"

Bruce: In a minute, but right now it's important that we let Diana have her time. I know it's hard, but she needs to feel what she feels, and I need to be here with her.

Dave: Yeah, me too!

And so the group sat with Diana and watched her cry.

As Diana was preparing for her discharge from the hospital, she reminded me of that session. She told me that it was important for her, but what had really made the difference that day was that I had not gotten into a "scene" with Dave. She said, "I decided that if you could be nice to him with what he drew, it would be okay for me to talk about that stuff."

As art therapists we work with images that come from the innermost parts of ourselves and our patients. I do not believe that it is an overstatement to describe this work as an act of love. In fact, it may be an understatement to define it as anything less than love. The doing of art, and of therapy requires great effort. Both actions call for self-transcendence and challenge human inertia. The facing of this challenge for the sake of the patient and for one's self is an act of love and courage.

As I stand before the chalk-smeared paper and see what my patient has done, I attend to her story. I am awed by her work, her courage and the love that encircles patient and therapist, artist and image.

Love is the will to attend. This is an essential concept that must be shouted within the halls of higher education.

Chapter XX

THE ROLE OF ASSESSMENT

In the midsummer of 1988 I became part of a long-range planning task force with a two-fold charge: 1) to design an environment for the short-term hospitalization of children and adolescents aged four to seventeen years; 2) to outline the services, both evaluative and treatment, and how they would be delivered. Harding Hospital had made a commitment to develop a "state of the art program" and to build a new facility to contain it.

A recurrent concern of the task force in its weekly meetings was how we could provide thorough evaluative workups in a very short time. We assumed that the length of stay would be less than one month for most of our prospective patients. In fact, we attempted to design programmatic components that could be fully implemented in two weeks or less. The time frame presented a challenge for psychological and neurological testing. In order to provide a complete diagnostic and treatment-oriented assessment, the psychology department usually required several weeks to complete the battery of tests and generate the written summary report. The clinician's written report is always of the highest quality, but the task force feared that it would do little good in terms of planning hospital treatment if the report came post-discharge. Further, there was often a waiting list for psychological testing. We imagined patients being referred for testing on the day of admission, but never actually being tested. This was not acceptable for a short-term, crisis intervention and evaluation unit.

I proposed that we consider using an art therapy assessment process, both as an initial evaluative procedure and as a screen for selecting patients who clearly needed the full battery of psychological tests. My suggestion got a warm reception, particularly when I said I felt an assessment could be administered routinely within 48 hours of admission to the unit, and a complete written report made available to the treatment team within another 48 hours. In response to concerns expressed by the representative of the psychology department on the task force, I assured her that in no way would art assessments duplicate psychological services, nor would the art therapists violate the professional boundaries of another discipline (Fig. 17).

With the full endorsement of the short-term task force, my colleague, Deb DeBrular, and I began to explore the existing art therapy assessment literature. Many of the assessment tools we reviewed seemed to be attempts to standardize artistic procedures. We did not think this direction would be helpful. Remembering Shaun McNiff's admonition, we didn't want to become *clever interpreters,* nor did we wish to create a *formula* approach to imaginal symbolism. We had no use for a systemtatized assessment procedure in which snakes always equaled penises and caves were always vaginas.

The more we defined what art therapy assessments should *not* be, we saw more clearly just what we wanted them to be. We wanted to provide the treatment team with a glimpse of the inner life of the patient-in-crisis. It could be said that we wanted to create a way to take a candid snapshot of the psyche/soul: not standardized, measurable data, but fleeting peeks at interior worlds.

We isolated eleven aspects of art processes that we felt would provide the art therapist with enough clues to be able to construct a thorough, reliable narrative description of the patient's sense of self, world view and relationship to others. It was intended as an outline, not a checklist. I have strong reservations about the use of checklists in mental health systems. They seem to reduce a complex human being, who happens to be a patient, to a convenient read-out of observed behaviors. My objection is on ethical and moral grounds. No human being should be reduced to dots, circles or checks on computer data sheets or medical records database forms. Attempts to summarize a person's strengths, weaknesses, motives and pathologies should require the concentrated effort of narrative form.

Our outline took shape:

MEDIA. We focused first on the use of media. A variety of media options, with different material qualities, should be provided for the patient's choice.

Examples:

——————————— **CONTINUUM** ———————————

resistive
(charcoal)

pliable
(Play-doh®)

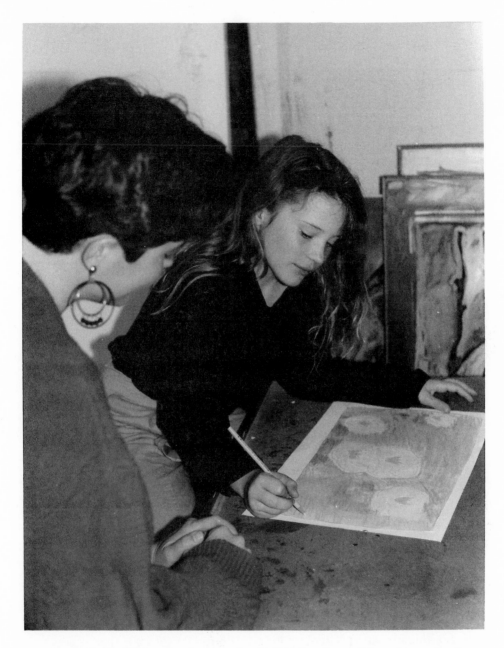

Figure 17. We didn't want to become what McNiff describes as, "clever interpreters."

_____ CONTINUUM _____

controllable	fluid
(pencils)	(water colors)
familiar	unfamiliar
(crayons)	(oil pastels)
meticulous-fine motor	gross motor
(pen and ink)	(tempera paint)
(fine brush)	(wide sponge applicator)

We sensed that attentiveness to media characteristics and the patient's selection process would provide a key to understanding the patient, not in isolation but in conjunction with other focal areas.

MOTION. The second area of attention is to the motions used by the patient during the assessment interview. Here again there is a spectrum of possibilities.

Examples:

_____ CONTINUUM _____

tight/constricted	loose/fluid
rythmic	spasmodic
fine	gross
aggressive	passive

It was our sense that patients, given the anxiety of being newly hospitalized, would select in the assessment situation motions with which they are most comfortable, and in an entirely non-verbal way would offer hints about their usual styles of coping with, or defending against anxiety.

PROCEDURES. A third focal area was procedures. We wondered what patients might tell us about themselves through the procedural aspects of a freely-chosen task. Would they choose tasks that require a degree of motor and mental coordination? Would they choose tasks that involved an element of technical awareness, or would simple repetitive tasks be preferred? What is their level of procedural competence? Does the patient invest in learning new skills in the midst of the session, or does he or she rely on familiar processes? We felt the answers to these kinds of questions would help in the assessment.

SYMBOL. Fourth, we wanted to pay close attention to the symbolic language of the patient. In some ways, this is the most difficult of the focal areas, since it clearly opens the door to evaluator projection. Still, the underlying premise of the arts therapies, that everything we create is a self-portrait, implies that there is a wealth of information in the imaginal symbolic creations of the patient. We had to rely on the subjective wisdom of the assessor. It was hoped that the symbols inherent in imagery, when presented in the context of all the other focal areas, would provide a rich portrait of the patient's inner world.

We made note that not only the created images are symbolic, but also the procedures, media, tools, physical motions, postures and verbalizations may represent unconscious needs, drives, perceptions and feelings.

SEXUAL IDENTIFICATION. The fifth focal area is sexual identification. In this perspective we make note of the patient's choice of task, style of implementation, interactive style and image content. Attention is paid to the frame of reference. Are all these factors typically associated with masculinity or femininity? Is the artist's style of engagement with the task best described as passive, fine, intricate or delicate? Or is it more aggressive, resistive and rough? The assessor is asked to make symbolic associations in the context of the overall assessment process.

SELF–INDULGENCE. The sixth area of focus might best be described as *degree* of self-indulgence. Does the patient derive pleasure from the exhibitionistic aspect of this process? Does she employ her own creative energy in the task or is her response mechanical, without narcissistic pleasure? Does he value the end product and wish to take it with him, or does he abandon it without comment at the end of the session?

DEPENDENCE/INDEPENDENCE. The seventh area is the continuum of dependent/independent action. Does the patient enjoy or flourish under the nebulous expectation, "create whatever you want?" or does he demand in one form or another to be structured by the assessor? Does the patient exhibit unique, individual performance? Does she identify with the end product as an expression of self? Are references made to her own body image or level of competencies?

ARTISTIC DEVELOPMENTAL LEVEL. The eighth focal area is that of artistic developmental level. For this, we chose to use the developmental categories outlined by Viktor Lowenfeld (*) We felt that Lowenfeld's work was based most clearly on a developmental model of health rather than pathology and would provide the evaluator with a normalized frame of reference.

LITERAL DESCRIPTION. The ninth category is a very literal exploration of what the patient creates. In this we attempt to pay attention to the shapes, lines, textures and colors without attaching any symbolic meaning.

FEELING TONE. The tenth focal area is that of the overall feeling tone of a given image. Again this depends upon the assessor's ability to be open to the image. One might describe this as an exercise in informed objective emotional responsiveness.

SUBJECTIVE RESPONSE. The final focus of the art assessment is the subjective response of the assessor. The assessor must apply the disciplines of looking, listening, being with and monitoring internal reactions.

The art therapy assessment can be summarized as follows:

attention to media *plus*
attention to motion *plus*
attention to procedures *plus*
attention to symbols *plus*
attention to sexual identification *plus*
attention to self indulgence *plus*
attention to dependence/independence *plus*
attention to artistic developmental level *plus*
attention to literal description *plus*
attention to feeling tone *plus*
attention to subjective response

EQUALS. Raw data of the narrative report.

This is not an easy process. The art therapy assessment procedure is quite time consuming. Generally it requires an hour to administer the assessment with the patient, an additional hour to organize and outline the report and roughly two hours to write the narrative.

It must be stressed that the writing of the narrative demands good basic writing skills. The assessor must not only be able to administer and organize the data, but then must present it clearly. Solid grammar, vocabulary and sentence and paragraph construction skills are necessary.

The art therapy assessment can offer psychiatric treatment teams a unique view of the patient. To be respected by other professionals it must be presented professionally. It is essential that training programs provide students with ample practical experience in media, observation, developmental psychology, outline and articulation.

The narrative report is outlined as follows:

I. Introduction
    A. describe the initial encounter
    B. describe the patient's general behavioral response

II. Analysis of symbol, media and emotional tone
  A.–K. review the eleven focal areas
III. Summary
  A. overview of the assessment
  B. treatment implications

EXAMPLE:

Art Therapy Assessment Interview Report

Stephen _____

Introduction

Stephen _____, a 14-year-old caucasian male, was seen for an art therapy assessment interview December 2, 1990. He presented himself as a pleasant, compliant, relatively easy to engage young man. He was fairly comfortable with the tasks presented to him and he approached the art processes with enthusiasm. His motions, however, were constricted throughout the interview.

As the art media were explained to him and offered for use, Stephen was hesitant. He stated that he is not good with paint and that he was unfamiliar with several of the other media available. After four or five minutes of perservation, he chose to work with pencil on an 18″ × 24″ piece of white paper. Despite his hesitancy in choosing materials, he appeared to derive gratification from using "such a big piece of paper." He commented three times that he wished he could have paper like this to draw on at home.

When given the opportunity to freely choose his subject matter for drawing, Stephen again was hesitant. This interviewer reassured him several times that whatever he chose to draw would be acceptable. After three to four minutes of silent inactivity, Stephen looked to the interviewer and requested that I give him an idea. After attempting once again to support free choice, to no avail, I suggested that he draw a tree that would symbolize himself. He began to work immediately and seemed to relax within the structure.

Analysis of Media, Symbols and Emotional Tone

When offered a variety of artistic materials, Stephen seemed overwhelmed. He was hesitant to utilize media with which he was unfamiliar.

After several minutes of consideration, he chose to work with a standard #2 pencil on white paper. This may be significant in several ways: 1) the pencil is the most highly controllable of all the media options; 2) the pencil is the most common and familiar of the media; 3) the pencil is the most limited in that it has no color and can be erased if perceived mistakes are made; 4) pencil is the least subject to accident or spontaneous utilization. When these media characteristics are coupled with Stephen's tight and constricted range of motion, one begins to glimpse the inhibition he experiences internally.

The image that Stephen created is an intriguing one. The tree is depicted as a large hickory. It was too large to be contained by the paper. He stated that this tree reminded him of one that grows in a field near his home. He portrayed a large, sturdy trunk which runs off the page. About halfway up the trunk a network of branches emerges. On the trunk, below the branch system, he drew a thick poison ivy vine which wraps around the trunk. Stephen devoted much time and energy to rendering the branches and the poison ivy realistically. However, the base of the trunk, where it meets the ground, is drawn in a minimalist and stylized fashion. The ground line is depicted with a single wavy line, roughly three inches above the bottom of the page. Significantly, the ground line does not extend from edge to edge on the paper. This is in contrast to both the trunk and the branch system, which as noted earlier both run off the page. This may indicate Stephen's sense that his foundation is not secure. This is further validated by the absence of any visual references to a root system. When commenting upon this, Stephen said, "I guess there are no roots."

Stephen's drawing style is fairly advanced, and he is technically a skilled renderer. In looking at his style of application of pencil to paper, one is struck by the effort and clarity with which he portrayed the branches and ivy, when contrasted with the very light, faint and sketchy handling of the lower trunk and ground surface.

In the branch system itself, it is interesting that he drew a complex system of thick, solid-looking limbs and myriad small twig-like sub-branches. Literally there are a hundred or more of these small, carefully detailed branches.

The tree is depicted standingby itself in an open field. No other trees are in view and no other life forms are shown. The overall emotional impact of this image is a sense of loneliness, isolation and abandonment.

There are multiple symbols inherent in this piece. One may certainly view Stephen's attention to detail in the branches as indicative of his interest in reaching out into the world. The branch system dominated his use of time and clearly was the area of most interest to him. The image is complicated, suggesting that for Stephen the appropriate developmental task of reaching outward toward others, particularly peers, is a complex yet crucial matter for him.

The trunk of the tree is raather paradoxical. On the one hand it appears to be a strong, thick trunk, while on the other hand he drew it in a sketchy and tentative manner. In addition, the trunk is encircled by poison ivy, which appears to be suffocating or constricting it.

The root system is non-existant and the trunk fades into the ground. As roots tend to represent nourishment and attachment, this image suggests a detached, malnourished view.

As he worked, Stephen spontaneously associated this tree with the cultural reference, a family tree. He mentioned several different members of his immediate and extended family. Through several vignettes, he shared his belief that his family has always regarded him as defective. He stated that his parents used to say he had "spells," which they referred to as "fits and fevers." Other vignettes he shared revolved around what he described as "funny things" that happen at family reunions when everybody drinks too much.

Stephen also spoke of times when he has been at the real tree that his drawing represents. He shared warm feelings and memories of playing on or around the tree when he was a child. He indicated that these were usually times when he was by himself and happy.

The recurrent metaphoric themes connected with this image would seem to be four-fold. The first is the sketchy, faint manner in which the tree is connected (or unconnected) with the ground. This indicates a sense of detachment and feelings of abandonment. Second, the poison ivy wrapped around the tree suggests his sense of being *damaged goods*. Third, the branch system on which he exerted such focused effort may represent the interest and energy Stephen utilizes toward the end of connecting with others. Finally, the tree is drawn in the season of winter. There are no leaves shown at all and one is left with a sense of bleak depression.

Summary

Stephen presents himself as a young man who is pleasant, yet depressed and isolated. He possesses above average artistic skills and this is an area of strength. He is particularly adept in visual abstract processing. This is in contrast to his view of self as inadequate, especially in relation to school performance. This suggests that his underlying feelings of self-loathing and abandonment disrupt his ability to function at age appropriate life tasks.

In relation to his treatment it will be important for treaters to pay attention to Stephen's discomfort in peer socialization situations. This is an area in which he feels quite inadequate and he may benefit from therapeutic activities that promote the development of communication and relating skills. While he can superficially appear pleasant and enjoyable, treaters must remain aware of his perception of himself as being *damaged goods.*

Another area of strength for Stephen is his ability to work in a concentrated manner for a fairly lengthy period. He stayed on task and worked intently for forty-five minutes. This suggests a capacity to focus in areas that interest him.

For successful treatment to occur, it will be imperative that attention be given to his view of the family. The vignettes he shared regarding family interactions and his sense of place indicate problematic relating styles.

Treaters will also want to give attention to Stephen's areas of strength. Visual tasks and other related activities may be gratifying to him. Such activities may also serve to loosen his constricted movement style and build his sense of competence and mastery in the world. These experiences will be given additional meaning if Stephen receives validation from significant others.

Bruce L. Moon, M.Div., A.T.R.

The information and suggestions provided by the art assessment were translated into a dynamic hospital treatment plan by the psychiatric team. A regimen of activities therapies was prescribed, including a Communication Skills Group, Adolescent Creative Activity and Physical Education/Recreation Group. In addition, he and his family were entered into intensive family therapy.

The team did not feel, based on this report, that individual psychotherapy was indicated at the present time.

Chapter XXI

THE ROLE OF HISTORY

In the clinical setting the need for a personal history of the patient has been well-established. In particular, patients suffering from Borderline Personality Disorder and Post Traumatic Stress Disorder exemplify the essential nature of ties to the past. Without a sense of connection to what has been, it is nearly impossible for the patient to be clear and stable with what is in the present and may be yet to come in the future. These diagnostic categories carry with them a pervasive phenomenon of a *historicity,* whether through developmental dysfunction or traumatic disruption.

In *Existential Art Therapy,* I offered the illustration of Donna, an a historical borderline adolescent.[3] In her case the primary task of the treatment team was to help her create a past, through the use of art and the establishment of positive relationships. In commenting upon the role of the arts in this historical creation, Dr. Robert Huestis, Director of the Department of Psychiatry at Harding Hospital, said, "These (the art images) are the windows that the patients allow us to look through as they struggle to create a past so they can function in the future, rather than live only in the present."[3]

The wisdom in Dr. Huestis's words goes beyond the clinical relevance to particular patients. When it is applied to the profession of creative arts therapy, we can glimpse the root of the identity confusion that is present today. The art therapy profession is, in some degree, ahistorical. We lack systematic recounting of our disciplinary development. To be sure, over the years at national conferences of the American Art Therapy Association there have been presentations that serve to some degree to tell the story of our birth and growth. The problem with this tradition, as with others, is that the events and their meanings are colored by the interpretation of the speaker. I have heard the pioneers tell their versions of the history. The stories often conflict. Some argue that art therapy began on the east coast; others contend that Kansas, or California or Austria has rightful claim as the birthplace. There may be truth in each of these claims. Certainly any history of art therapy must include the names of Florence Cane, Margaret Naumberg, Elinor Ulman, Don Jones, Myra Levick, Janie Rhyne, Edith Kramer, Arthur Robbins, Bob Ault, Mary Huntoon, Felice Cohen and many others. All of these, and more, made significant contributions at critical stages of our development.

It is important that creative arts therapy education programs make every effort to present as complete a history to our students as possible. Too often the history of the field has been a political platform from which one faction or another proclaimed its "truth." Perhaps it was inevitable, as the various giants of the profession vied for prestige and recognition. By now, most of the pioneers of the field have made peace with themselves and with one another. A definitive history of the profession must be written in the future. For now, programs must try to offer their students the broadest possible chronicle of the past. From this foundation, current students and practitioners may have a more solid sense of self as professionals, with a past, present and future.

Just as the ahistorical patient must develop a history in order to function today and tomorrow, our profession must be based upon the foundations laid by our pioneer predecessors.

The Creative Encounter

In an earlier section of this work, I commented on the necessary sense of history that helps form our identity as arts therapists. As is often the case when dealing with the complex, prismatic form of art and therapy processes, I will now turn attention to the opposite facet: the abandonment of past and future during the creative encounter. It is paradoxical that as I approach the canvas as an artist, or the patient as a therapist, I must bring all of my experience and knowledge to the encounter, and yet once there must let go of past biases or worries about the future in order to be genuinely in the present.

I have been known to be quite emphatic in my reprimand of students who lament that they failed to concentrate fully in the session with the patient because they were distracted by worries over car trouble they had earlier in the day. I am very firm as I tell the student, "You have no right to be distracted or preoccupied when in the company of your patient." It is essential that therapists be nowhere else than in the present when doing therapy. This may seem a harsh demand, but I believe it is a realistic and attainable goal.

In order to understand the nature of this intense *here and now* creative encounter, it is helpful to turn to the art process itself as a metaphor of the experience. The problem of the creative encounter may best be examined through the analogous observation of the artist in the inspirational phase of creative work. The artist loses all sense of past and future, existing only in the present moment. Totally absorbed, fascinated and immersed in the here and now task, the artist is *all there.*

The willingness and capacity to be locked into the present seems to be a fundamental attribute for creative action. It may be described as a loss of ego, or more positively as a transcendence of self. There is an integration, a fusion of sorts between the artist and the media. Regardless of media, paint, dance, music or rhyme, artists describe a sense of ecstatic revelation and bliss.

Don Jones describes these experiences as *epiphanies;* Abraham Maslow refers to them as *peak experiences.* Whether we regard them as natural psychological events or trans-human processes, the common characteristics seem to be a complete and compelling fascination with the task at hand. Such depictions of the focal processes of art have much to offer in enriching our understanding of the creative encounter with the patient. We need not, however, become enthralled with the art aspect of this phenomenon. All people have experienced similar circumstances in the normal course of life. Most people have become so absorbed in a good book or thrilling movie that they lose track of time. One can easily become lost in any task that is of great interest. Still, the creative state does serve as a clear illustration and I will use it here. Let us review the characteristics of what happens during these experiences:

The Artist. As the painter moves her brush from palette to canvas, she is aware that she has done the motions before. She is aware that she has used the medium before and perhaps employed the same color combinations in earlier work. In this sense her past is a part of her. It is assimilated throughout her being. Yet, she cannot paint again what she painted before. To try to do so would lead to frustration and estrangement from the work before her. She must give up the past, let it go, in order to be with the canvas that is now.

Joni Mitchell comments during a recorded concert (*Miles of Aisles*), "Nobody ever asked Van Gogh, paint *A Starry Night* again."

The Therapist. The arts therapist must similarly allow past encounters with patients to be in the current session only by way of being fully integrated, digested aspects of self. The intervention so effective with one depressed patient last week may have little or no therapeutic benefit to the depressed patient before him today.

Artist. As the painter works, she cannot afford to look too far ahead in the process. To do so would be to become oblivious to the emerging image in the present. The moment must be allowed to stand for its own sake, not solely as a springboard to some future process.

Therapist. The same is true within the therapeutic creative encounter. The therapist must attend to what the patient is doing now, rather than hypothesizing what might happen next session. In the existential sense there is no next session, there is only this one. In the realistic, pragmatic sense, there may be no next time. The therapist must be an agent for good in this moment.

Artist. As she paints, she works without guile, oblivious to what should, or ought, to be happening. The interaction between herself and the image dictates the moment, not some dogmatic rule. There is a sense of childlike naivete or purity of intent that may be likened to standing naked. She is receptive to the moment without manipulation or demand.

Therapist. I have often felt myself to be rather childlike and even foolish in the early stages of therapy. Often patients will test my intentions with defensive cruelty. Doing therapy is an opening of oneself, a making vulnerable to another, which is foolishness in the best sense. Within the therapeutic encounter, the therapist must bring an innocent positive regard for the other's well being.

Artist. Images form before her on the canvas and she is less aware of outside influences. She is focused fully on the canvas. The artist has abandoned her public facades, forgotten her desires to influence others, to gain recognition and win approval. Through the artistic process she is able to be herself, genuinely, authentically. With no distractions, she is able to attach herself completely to the task of painting.

Therapist. I usher the patient in and close the door to my private practice office. I can feel my masks begin to loosen. I take my customary position in the room and feel one of my masks fall away completely. My patient begins to draw and another pulls away from my face. For the next fifty minutes I have no audience, no one to act for, no one to please. With no script to read from and no theme to improvise from, I am free to be with my patient genuinely and devote myself to her drama.

Artist. Images continue to form. She is caught up in the birth within her and without. She does not critique or edit, she does not reject or judge, she just lets the paint flow.

Therapist. As the patient works I become absorbed in her process. I watch and be with. I do not cut her off, or analyze. I do not interpret or evaluate. I just let the session flow.

Artist. She steps back from the painting to get a broader look at the work in progress. She does not indulge in worrying what others will say about the piece. She does not censor the work for the sake of acceptance. There is an air of stubborn self-confidence. The necessary acceptance comes from within herself, not from without. It could be mistaken for arrogant self-sufficiency. In the creative moment there is an intrinsic uninhibited, defenseless, genuine quality. Fear and indecision have been forsaken, replaced by an inner strength and courage. Such artistic, self-absorbed courage allows the artist to be open to the mysterious, ambiguous and paradoxical. Courage paves the way to action.

Therapist. My patient, a fifteen-year-old adolescent girl, steps away from the image she has created. Tears slide down her cheeks. I look in awe at the scene of a little five-year-old girl being sodomized by a malevolent babysitter. I am horrified and appalled, but I must face this monstrous image with stubborn, open courage. If I show the slightest fear or repulsion, she may well misinterpret it as judgment of her. I will not indulge my fear. It is the enemy of creativity. For the moment I will be with this little girl and we will be strong and courageous together. We will look at this painful image with stubborn confidence. We will not be intimidated or sick anymore. Creative encounters banish fear.

Artist. Positive and optimistic, she picks up the brush again and moves back towards the canvas. She accepts the image that is being born. She lets it be itself, she is receptive and humble, she lets the process have its own way.

Therapist. As my patients slowly bring their traumatic images to the studio, unfolding themselves in paint or chalk or clay, I make every effort to approve and bring honor to the unfoldings. I maintain an attitude of awe in the company of patient artistry. I accept their offerings and in every way I can imagine, I ennoble them. Regardless of the visual form, I respond in the positive, affirming the validity of their creative struggle.

Artist. She paints, trusting the process. She waits, quietly receptive. Willing to forgo the desire to master and control, she trusts the process.

Therapist. Many times in my life, I have had problems with my characteristic need to feel dominant or in control. Excessive focus on mastery or technique has affected my golf swing, sexual performance, supervisory responsibilities and most certainly my therapy sessions. I have had to learn to relax and trust the process. I learned to float on my back in water as soon as I quit flailing about. Likewise I have become a much more effective art therapist since I abandoned my attempts to control the therapy. I trust the process.

Artist. Suddenly as she works, the grey-green bleeds into the burnt sienna. She watches the accident, then gently, instinctually works in concert with the unexpected. She did not intend for this to happen, but her capacity to adapt to the situation at hand allows her to use the accident in a positive, nearly effortless, intuitive way. She did not allow the bleeding to become a battleground.

Therapist. As art therapists we must allow ourselves to concentrate so completely upon the task before us, with such fascination and awe, that we can function spontaneously. Our competencies must promote flexibility as the situation demands, continuously adapting to the demands of the here-and-now encounter. As the waters of an ocean adapt to the continuously shifting contours of the shore, so we must be intuitive enough to flow with the process.

Creative arts therapy educators must provide an educational environment that promotes students' epiphanies, ecstasies and peak experiences. We must role model authentic engagement in the creative encounter. This must be a threepronged approach in the educational environment.

First, the teacher/supervisor/mentor must teach by example. The instructor must not only describe experiences to the class, but also provide opportunities for the individuals in the class to have such experience within the course context.

Second, educational programs must re-establish their link to art processes, which are the root of authentic being. Studio art must re-emerge as a requirement in masters level training programs.

Finally, students in the clinical setting must receive appropriate supervisory support that emphasizes the essential nature of the therapy hour as a creative encounter.

Chapter XXII

THE ROLE OF WORK

The farmer plows the earth, he harrows it, tears it,
pulverizes it; he pulls out weeds, or cuts them, or burns
them; he poisons insects, and fights against drought and
floods. To be sure, all of this is done in order to create
something, for which reason we can call it work and
not rage.[32]

Karl A. Menninger
LOVE AGAINST HATE, Chapter 6

Menninger's illustration could easily be expanded to include the ceramicist pounding and kneading of the clay, or the melting and pouring of metal into molds, or the mining and burning of coal for power. In each case it is the same: destructive force is used for constructive purposes, i.e., work.

You may wish to question this by offering examples of more passive occupational pursuits such as the computer programmer, the teacher, sales clerk. Yet in each case there is a significant motivating factor which, when looked at deeply, seems very close to the urge to master. The computer programmer seeks to organize, reformulate and control data. The teacher directs, shapes and molds the intellectual growth of her students. In each case, we grasp the underlying impulse to assert mastery over the environment.

It is no coincidence that work is often closely associated with the arts. When an exhibit is opened, the objects are described as *works of art*. They are not publicized as *plays* of art, they are works of art. It is curious, then, that in our current cultural viewpoint the arts are considered frivolous. In our public education system, the arts are often the first targets of budget cuts and are almost never offered on a daily basis as are mathematics and sciences. The arts have come to be viewed as something one does in leisure time, rather than one's work.

Our students bring to the educational setting a long history, both personal and cultural, of this paradox: on the one hand the notion of

153

artwork, and on the other hand a view of art as a *frill.* This presents a peculiar dilemma for the creative arts therapy educator: how to rediscover the *work* of art as a mindset within the novice therapist in order to enable the student to ennoble the work of the artist/patient?

The patient does not come to art psychotherapy in order to engage in frills-therapy. The patient comes to work on intra- and interpersonal difficulties. The therapist, regardless of benevolent intention, who view the arts as anything less than the transformation of destructive energy into constructive ends, will inevitably fail the patient. Such a therapist will fail to grasp the depth and significance of the work that lies ahead of the patient. The work will be falsely trivialized and the patient will ultimately be frustrated by the futility of the struggle. Compounding the problem, the therapist may fail to own the work he or she must do in the encounter: the reforming of destructive patterns and redefining the self-defeating resistances of the patient. This is hard work, neither trivial nor frilly.

In preparing art therapists, it is essential to engender a profound respect for the *work* of art, of the patient and of the therapist. The drive toward mastery is one of the strongest motivations in each of these three aspects of the work. The sense of competence derived from mastery of complicated problems is directly linked to self-discipline, which eventuates in pleasure. There grows from this what I would describe as a sacred passion for life. The sacred passion is marked by an authentic, creative and vital relationship between the individual and the world. Such experiences are intrinsically tied to the artist's use of media in a masterful way. Technical skill is empty without the emotional investment of the artist. The success of any art work depends not only on its communication of feeling, but also upon its demonstration of competent handling of materials.

The art therapist must not rely solely upon the transitory cathartic expression of the patient, but must also consider the influence of formal artistic techniques on the expression. As arts therapists are trained, there must be careful attention given to ongoing development of their grasp of arts processes, hand in hand with relationship skills, communication skills and psychotherapeutic technique.

In the most profound sense, mastery may be viewed as the capacity to organize and transform experience. When we couple this view with the previously mentioned description of work, we arrive at a formulation of the significance that art work manifests in psychotherapeutic work: engagement in art tasks provides a therapeutic milieu in which powerful destructive forces are transformed into constructive, meaningful objects. Art organizes chaotic emotional experience and gives the artist a coherent, reorganized product. It is the swirling mix of feelings, sensations, actions and relationships that are the markers of emotional and mental distress. The arts, at a metaverbal level, gradually serve to alleviate the distress through the work itself, by providing hope for clarity and balance.

As the patient's sense of competence builds in relation to a particular artistic task, there is invariably a corresponding increase in the individual's self-esteem and confidence. This establishes a reciprocity between artist/patient, task and product that is cross-contagious. As the artist grows in ability to handle material, the ability to handle other aspects of life grows as well, and vice-versa.

Having said that, I am compelled to caution the reader that technical competence itself will not alleviate the dysfunction of the patient. Were that the case there would be no need for arts therapists, but only art teachers. My intent is only to highlight one specific aspect of the prismatic nature of our field, which, in my view, has too often been forsaken in pursuit of expression. Form and function are essential to each other, as are tragedy and opportunity in the Chinese proverb, different sides of the same coin.

Over the past several decades the notion of work has undergone an intriguing developmental schism that is worth comment as it relates to the training and education of students of arts therapies. A significant segment of the population has grown to view work as drudgery that must be endured for forty hours a week. It is almost as if employment is the sentence for the crime of growing up. Many popular and country ballads have poeticized the sentiment: "You can take this job and shove it."[33]

Another view of work is typified by the *workaholic,* the person who cannot separate himself from his work, who is in essence addicted to the job. These are the individuals who log sixty, seventy or more hours on the job each week; who eat, sleep and live their professions, perhaps because there is little else of meaning in their lives.

A third view is a hedonistic perspective in which the work is seen purely as a means to an end, the end being material gain. This category is best represented by the young urban professional (*yuppie*) who stereotypically measures the meaning of his life in objects and appliances synonymous with success.

It is increasingly difficult to find individuals who manifest a well-balanced and positive view of their employment situation, their work. I believe in the truism that actions speak louder than words. It is not too much of an intellectual leap to suggest that what we do is what we are. For most adults in our culture, what we do for much of our lives is our work, therefore our work largely defines who we are.

It is tragic that so many individuals define themselves as prisoners, or addicts, or hedonists. Creative arts therapy students, having lived in this culture, will bring to the training situation one of these views of work, in one form or another. It is essential that educational systems and teachers be attentive to these possibilities. By focusing on an artistic understanding of work, programs can do much to help the student develop a healthier perspective. Value questions must be raised in a variety of forms: didactically, in dialogue and through active studio work.

The development of a healthy, balanced and meaning-filled attitude about work cannot only be taught, it must be modeled by the teacher, mentor, supervisor. Failing to do this will have an effect upon future patients. The therapist who subtly views his work as enslavement can hardly free the patient from chaos. The therapist who is overly committed, addicted to the work will no doubt leak his compulsion into the therapy milieu. The therapist who is much concerned with his own material gain will find it nearly impossible to discover meaning in the broken, ruined or disfigured aspects of the patient's self-image. For the good of all future patients it is essential that positive values about the nature of work be fostered and nourished in the academic program.

Chapter XXIII

PAINTING MY WAY HOME

For a little more than a year I worked with our clinical interns in the painting studio. I was teaching a course titled *Studio Methods Seminar*. Its stated purpose is to place the student in the creative arts studio without the distractions of patient responsibilities. The focus is ongoing creative self-exploration and development of the professional value of maintaining one's own artistic development. The student is provided with an opportunity to integrate, through the artistic process, the wide range of academic, clinical and emotional experiences inherent in graduate art therapy study. The core expectation is that each student will work on major artistic pieces designed to integrate the internship experience. It is expected that each student will complete no fewer than five major works during the program.

The seminar meets for one and one-half hours per week. Generally students are expected to finish one piece every three months. These works may be paintings, sculptures, collage or other media that lend themselves to prolonged involvement. Evaluation is made based upon attendance, engagement with the task and completion of the works in a timely manner. Content of the work is a subject for discussion with the instructor, peers and the primary supervisor.

In addition to the stated purposes as outlined above, I now believe that there are other less observable, subtler objectives.

Several years ago my wife and I built our home. It is a 2,000 square foot log cabin. It is safe to say that 95 percent or more of every piece of wood in the house bears our fingerprints. I recall many instances during the five months of active construction, when my children, aged three and six at the time, sat and watched what we were doing. I thought then that they were hungry for parental attention, so they stayed close to us. While that is surely true, I have wondered since if they were not engaged in a research task. That is, they were studying Mom and Dad, making careful notes about what it is to be a man and a woman; what it is to work hard and what it is to create something as large as a house. In post-industrial America the opportunities for children to have such an extended laboratory experience of watching their parents is rare.

In the 1940s, 50s, 60s, the father dropped out of his children's view. He went to work, stayed there eight to twelve hours and came home tired. The economic and life style pressures of the 1970s, 80s and 90s have now extended this phenomenon to mothers as well. The stay-at-home housewife/mother is a rarity.

Our children learned many life lessons watching Cathy and me in a way that children have done for most of humankind's history.

Robert Bly writes of the absence of such experiences, "Not seeing your father when you are small, never being with him, having a remote father . . . is an injury."[34] Bly encourages men to re-engage in initiatory experiences between the generations.

The time I spend in studio with my students is initiatory ritual time. The primitive societies maintained that boys and girls could become men and women only through ritual and effort, and only with the active involvement of older men and women. This is true of the world of the art therapist as well. Young women and men do not enter the world of the arts therapist simply by taking the right courses. The active intervention of mentors is essential. This means that older practitioners must welcome and be with the novice who is entering the mythologized, intuitive world of the art therapy profession.

I regard the art therapy that I do as sacred. Each time a patient baptizes his wounds with paint or chalk, he receives the nourishment and courage his journey requires. Initiation in this sense does not mean rising above the pain, nor clinging to it; the therapy process (learning process) is found in knowing when and how to immerse oneself in the creative flow, in the presence of the mentor.

Much of the unspoken benefit of the Studio Methods Seminar for my students (and me) comes from this initiatory rite. I do not have to tell them that I believe in the power of the creative process. They can see my faith with their own eyes. I do not have to share verbally my concern that many art therapists quit doing art, for they will smell my sweat and commitment. They do not have to wander fearfully and alone through their journey, because I will stand with them and they will be welcomed into the ritual space.

Some may read this and insist that I am describing nothing more than role modeling. I want to be absolutely clear that while role modeling it is, it is so very much more. Ritual is myth/metaphor translated into action. The initiation ritual of our painting or working together is a significantly deeper process than role modeling could ever be.

Ritual in Progress

In April of 1991 I began a painting in Studio Methods Seminar (Fig. 18). I started by painting the entire canvas a light greenish blue. This was rather odd for me, since I seldom use pastel colors and only occasionally work with cool colors. My students commented that this was an "out of character" start. Regardless, something in the color seemed to call to me and I responded.

Then, having a solid pastel blue green square completed, I began work on the image of a table. I had no formal plan for this painting at all. I simply let it lead me where it wanted to go. When I finished the base color for the table, it looked so dark and heavy against the light background, it made me feel uncomfortable. I didn't want to look at it.

When I returned to the studio the following week, I was again repelled by the darkness of the table shape. I decided to cover part of the shape with a soft printed cloth. The image of a flowered table runner presented itself and was painted in. I was working on this section, I began thinking about my mother's house. My mother was eighty years old at the time and her house was filled with soft things—doilies and memorabilia of children, grandchildren and great-grandchildren. During this period of reflection it dawned on me that the painting might be a sort of nostalgia piece for me. I decided to hang (paint) a mirror on the left upper section of the canvas to emphasize this reflecting.

The moment I began to paint the frame of the mirror, I knew that the image it reflected should be of the kitchen in the house where I grew up. Suddenly the initial background color made sense.

"It's aqua," I said. My students looked at me with puzzlement.

"It's aqua. My sisters and I used to give my mom a hard time about always painting her kitchen the same color . . . aqua!"

The images in the mirror came quickly. The old porcelain sink, a dishrag hanging on the cabinet door. Violets on the window sill. A circular fluorescent light glaring from the ceiling. Kitchen table, cup of coffee, lit Chesterfield cigarette. These images are burned deeply into my memory of childhood (Fig. 19).

At some point one of my interns asked if I planned to paint a portrait

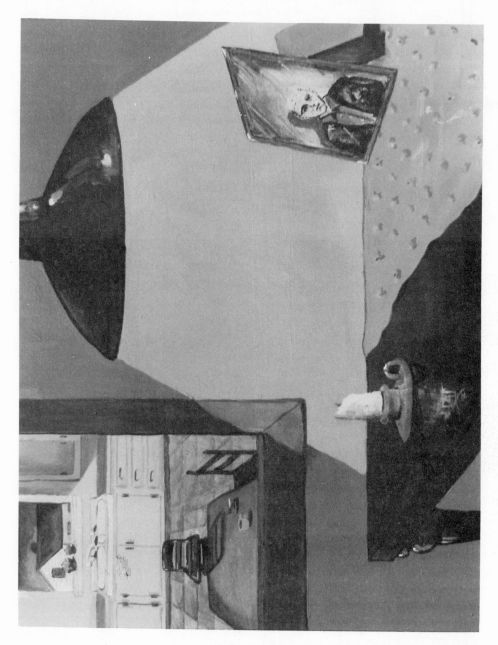

Figure 18. The initiation ritual of painting together is deeper than role modeling.

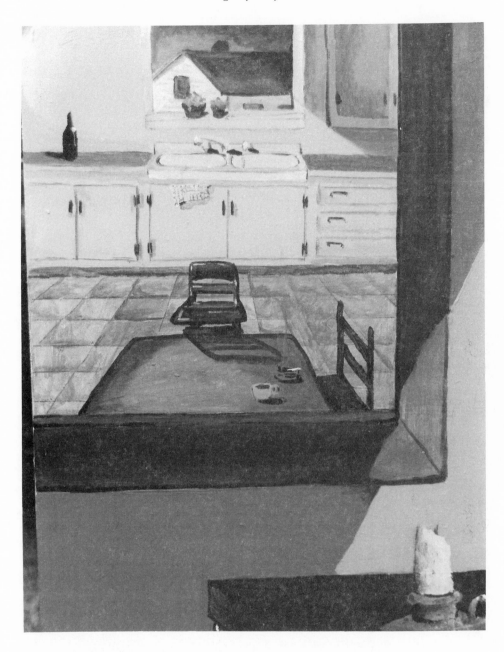

Figure 19. These images are burned deeply into my memory.

of my mother standing in the kitchen. I said that I wasn't sure, but something moved deep in the pit of my stomach as I answered.

I decided to move back to the table and avoid the kitchen for a time. Again, the images presented themselves quickly. I painted the candle and holder, but was unclear whether to paint a flame on the wick of the candle. The picture on the table was at first a portrait of my father as a young man. It portrayed him as a baseball catcher about to catch a fast ball.

A week went by.

When I returned to the studio the image of my father felt wrong. It's hard to describe. I just knew it was wrong. I painted over that section in white. Now the image of my father as a 44-year-old man (shortly before his death) emerged. This time the image felt good (Fig. 20).

One of my students commented, "Well, if you're going to have your dad in there, I think you'd better put your mother in the mirror." Again I was confronted with the issue.

The Studio Methods Seminar met every Wednesday afternoon from 3:30 till 5:00. On the Tuesday before the next session, July 16, I received an emergency phone call from my sister, telling me that Mother had had a serious stroke and the doctor wanted the immediate family to gather to discuss treatment options.

Over the next four weeks, my mother endured paralysis, inability to speak, hospitalization and transfer to a nursing home. She died on August 18, 1991.

As I entered the studio and looked at my nearly completed painting, its messages were clear and strong. This painting was a preparation of sorts for my mother's death. My struggle with whether to include her in the piece was an intuitive painful ritual of transition for me. I am now no one's son. I have no parents.

Arlene Weiss said to me, "You are a grown up orphan."

Yes.

The painting knew. I signed it on Wednesday, August 26, the ritual complete. My students watched this. They walked with me. They cannot doubt that I believe in the process. They have seen me dip my wounds in paint and draw the nourishment and strength I need to continue the journey. They have seen me paint my way home.

I welcome them.

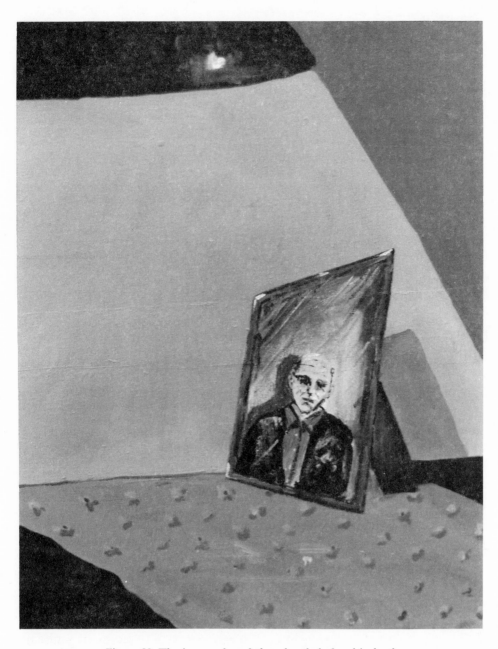

Figure 20. The image of my father shortly before his death.

EPILOGUE

Our journey together is nearly complete. We have traveled a path filled with images: images of mastery, beginning, chaos and order. I hope that through it all you have sensed the deep respect and passion I have for this art therapy profession of ours. There is really nothing I would rather do with my life (except maybe play professional basketball ... but, oh well). I have tried to present the reader with what I consider to be the essentials of the field. I worry that as we continue to evolve professionally we will allow others to define who and what we are. We have deep roots. It is my strongest wish that these remain the source of our nourishment.

Whether you are a teacher, student or practitioner in the creative arts therapies, I urge you always to keep the wonder, the mystery and the love of art before you and within you.

Yes, Peace ...
Bruce L. Moon

BIBLIOGRAPHY

1. Hillman, James, *A Blue Fire,* New York: Harper and Row, 1989.
2. Whyte, David, *Where Many Rivers Meet,* Langley, WA: Many Rivers Press, 1990.
3. Moon, Bruce, *Existential Art Therapy: The Canvas Mirror,* Springfield, IL: Charles C Thomas, 1990.
4. McNiff, Shaun, Lecture, Harding Hospital, Worthington, Ohio, 1991.
5. Janson, H.W., *History of Art,* New York: Harry N. Abrams, 1971.
6. Hopper, Edward, *Nighthawks,* 1942.
7. Moon, Catherine, Dialogue, 1991.
8. Kirkegaard, Soren, *Purity of Heart, To Will One Thing,* New York: Harper & Row, 1956.
9. Powers, Mary Lou, Unpublished Journal.
10. Webster's *New World Dictionary, Third College Edition,* New York: Simon and Schuster, 1988.
11. Selle, Joan, Unpublished Journal.
12. Kafka, Franz, *The Castle,* New York: Modern Library, 1954, 1969.
13. Frankl, Viktor, *Man's Search For Meaning: An Introduction to Logotherapy,* Philadelphia: Washington Square Press, 1969.
14. Mc Niff, Shaun, *Depth Psychology of Art,* Springfield, IL: Charles C Thomas, 1989.
15. Wadeson, Harriet, *Art Psychotherapy,* New York: John Wiley, 1980.
16. Feder & Feder, *Expressive Arts Therapies.* Englewood Cliffs, NJ: Prentice-Hall, 1981.
17. Guidelines For Academic, Institute and Clinical Art Therapy Training. Mundelein, IL: American Art Therapy Association, 1989.
18. Hillman, James, *ReVisioning Psychology,* New York: Harper & Row, 1975.
19. Campbell, Joseph, *The Power of Myth,* New York: Doubleday, 1988.
20. Rubin, Judith, *The Art of Art Therapy,* New York: Bruner Mazel, 1984.
21. Papini, Giovanni. A Visit to Freud. Reprinted in *Review of Existential Psychology and Psychiatry 9,* n.2, 1969.
22. Paxton, Tom, The Marvelous Toy, The Compleat Tom Paxton LP, New York: Deep Fork Music, Elektra Music, 1970.
23. DeBrular, Debra & Moon, Bruce, Precious Gifts, Unpublished paper, 1989.
24. Sillitoe, Allan, *The Loneliness of a Long Distance Runner,* New York: Signet/New American Library, 1959.
25. Nelson, James B., *Male Sexuality and Masculine Soirituality,* SIECUS Report, Vol. XIII Number 4, New York: The Sex Information and Education Council of the U.S., 1985.

26. Chowdorow, N., *The Reproduction of Mothering.* Berkley: University of California Press, 1978.
27. Dulicai, Hays, Nolan, Training the Creative Arts Therapist: Identity with Integration. *Arts and Psychotherapy, Vol. 16,* 1989.
28. Nietzsche, Frederich, As Quoted by Viktor Frankl, *Man's Search For Meaning: An Introduction to Logotherapy,* Philadelphia: Washington Square Press, 1953.
29. Stratford Philosophy Committee, Philosophy of Treatment Manual, Unpublished. Edited by Dr. Robert Huestis.
30. Simon, Paul, I Am A Rock, Sounds of Silence LP, New York: Eclectic Music, Columbia, 1965.
31. Peck, Scott, *The Road Less Traveled,* New York: Simon and Schuster, 1978.
32. Menninger, Karl, Love Against Hate.
33. Paycheck, Johnny, You Can Take This Job and Shove It, Warner-Tamerlane, 1977.
34. Bly, Robert, *Iron John,* New York: Addison-Wesley, 1990.

INDEX